SECOND EDITION

An Introduction to Research
for
MIDWIVES

For my wife, Brenda
and my sons, Michael and David

For Books for Midwives:

Senior Commissioning Editor: Mary Seager
Development Editor: Catharine Steers
Project Manager: Samantha Ross
Design Direction: George Ajayi

SECOND EDITION

An Introduction to Research for MIDWIVES

COLIN REES BSc(Econ) MSc(Econ) PGCE(FE)
Lecturer, University of Wales College of Medicine,
School of Nursing and Midwifery Studies,
Cardiff, Wales

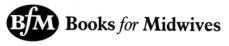 **Books** *for* **Midwives**

Edinburgh London New York Oxford Philadelphia St Louis Sydney Toronto 2003

BOOKS FOR MIDWIVES
An imprint of Elsevier Science Limited

First edition 1997
Second edition 2003

ISBN 0 7506 5351 5

British Library Cataloguing in Publication Data
A catalogue record for this book is available from the British Library

Library of Congress Cataloging in Publication Data
A catalog record for this book is available from the Library of Congress

Notice
Medical knowledge is constantly changing. Standard safety
precautions must be followed, but as new research and clinical
experience broaden our knowledge, changes in treatment and drug
therapy may become necessary or appropriate. Readers are advised to
check the most current product information provided by the
manufacturer of each drug to be administered to verify the recommended
dose, the method and duration of administration, and contraindications.
It is the responsibility of the practitioner, relying on experience and
knowledge of the patient, to determine dosages and the best treatment
for each individual patient. Neither the Publisher nor the author assume
any liability for any injury and/or damage to persons or property arising
from this publication.

The Publisher

**ELSEVIER
SCIENCE**
your source for books,
journals and multimedia
in the health sciences
www.elsevierhealth.com

The
publisher's
policy is to use
**paper manufactured
from sustainable forests**

Printed in China

Contents

Preface

At one time, if midwives read a research book, it indicated they were completing an assignment for a course. Now research is an accepted part of midwifery practice. This means we need to understand a range of research concepts and principles as part of evidence-based practice. One of the main barriers to using research, however, is 'the jargon', or worse, 'the statistics'. A further problem is that it is easy to forget some basic principles about research if you are not often drawing on that knowledge. One solution to these problems is a simple book on research that will act as an effective resource: a friend who will inform not intimidate.

This is what you are holding in your hands. The purpose of this book is to demystify research and make the subject accessible to midwives. The following chapters are designed to extend knowledge and develop a critical understanding of research in order to ensure evidence-based practice. It has been written in a simple, practical and purposeful way, so as to avoid reinforcing many people's worst fear that research is simply unintelligible jargon. If you should find any of the words confusing, there is a glossary of terms at the back of the book where you will find a clear explanation.

Although this book is a practical support for every midwife, it is particularly appropriate for anyone undertaking a course with a research component.

The book combines the following three themes:

1. Research methods and processes
2. The critical evaluation of research
3. The application of research to midwifery practice.

Each chapter outlines a key research topic and explains major issues that need consideration before applying research to practice. The relationship between the midwife and research is examined from two perspectives: first, the midwife as the 'doer' of research, that is, carrying out research, and second, the midwife as the 'user' of research, that is, critically assessing the research findings of others. Each role has different implications for the knowledge and skills required to achieve competence. These differences are clearly addressed at the end of each chapter under the heading 'Conducting research', which provides some practical advice on carrying out research, and 'Critiquing research', which outlines areas to consider when reading research reports. Each chapter ends with a list of key points that provide a summary of essential information.

Although textbooks are not meant to be read in a sequential order like a novel, Chapter 1 does start with a rationale for the importance of research in midwifery. Chapter 2 includes some fundamental concepts that will provide the groundwork for the remaining chapters, while Chapter 3 outlines the basic structure of research. Chapter 4 illustrates that research comes in a number of packages, and illustrates the relevance of qualitative research to midwifery. Once you have reached Chapter 5 on critiquing, the order in which you read the other chapters becomes less important. Reading is a personal activity, however, and you may find a different route through the book. If it is used as part of a course, you may use it more like a reference book and dip in at strategic points when a session or assignment necessitates. Whatever your reason for reading it, I hope you find it provides the answers to many of your questions about research and that it allows you to make better use of research in practice.

It is important to emphasize that this is an introduction to the extensive world of research. It is not meant to include chapters or sections on everything you may want to know about the subject. There are alternative resources that cover those topics in more depth, and these are indicated at appropriate points throughout the book. The topics that have been included are essential to an introduction to the subject. In particular, this book is built on the development of skills, not just the acquisition of knowledge. This approach has been used successfully over many years of teaching midwives, nurses and other health professionals. I hope you find it works for you.

Acknowledgements

I would like to express my gratitude first and foremost to Mary Seager at Elsevier, for supporting the idea of a second edition and for her patience while I slowly produced the goods.

I owe a great deal to the support and friendship of many midwifery educationalists who have believed in my ability to enthuse their students with a passion for research. In particular, I would like to thank Sandy Kirkman and Gail Williams in Cardiff, and Christine Tucker and Sheena Payne at the University of the West of England in Bristol.

Thank you to all the midwives and nurses who bought the first edition of the book, especially those I have had the pleasure to teach. Thanks in particular to the research module students whom I asked for ideas on how I could improve the first edition. I did what you suggested.

I would like to thank a special bunch of friends and work colleagues who have always supported me and who helped in producing this book. Thanks to Ian Hulatt, friend and best man, for some practical help, George McWhirter, for reading and making suggestions on the chapter on statistics, and to Jerry Bray, who always enthusiastically supports my work. I would also like to thank my longstanding friend Andy Mardell, who has provided practical support in helping me develop my research writing skills.

In producing this edition, as with the first, I have received so much practical and emotional support from my wife Brenda Rees, an inspirational Head of Midwifery. Her encouragement, enthusiasm and care made a huge difference. I have so much to thank her for and greatly appreciate everything she has done for me.

Finally, I would like to thank my two special sons, Michael and David Rees who have been so proud of my achievement in producing this book. I wish them every success with their futures.

Writing this second edition was probably more of a challenge than the first. I have attempted to continue the strength of the first edition by presenting research in a straightforward and down-to-earth style, and have extensively updated the referenced material. I believe research literacy is a crucial aspect of professional development. I hope this book helps you in making your personal contribution to your profession. Thank you.

CHAPTER ONE
Why Research?

Very few midwives would have difficulty in arguing why we need research. The continued advances in care and the maintenance of quality standards are both influenced by the amount of sound research available. Midwifery has always prided itself on the amount of research it undertakes, and the amount on which it draws. However, there have always been differences in the extent to which individual midwives made use of the latest research, and overall its use varied from clinical area to clinical area. This has meant that the standard of care can vary from midwife to midwife, and area to area. To overcome these differences there has been a concerted effort by the NHS to ensure all health professionals make better use of research, and to charge Trusts to support this through a structured approach to service provision.

This has been the role of Clinical Governance, which according to Miller (2002) provided a welcome focus for clinical improvement. It is a system that has brought about a change in the philosophy of service provision. Instead of health care organizations applying economic criteria to shape the delivery of care, the introduction of Clinical Governance in April 1999 made quality, as well as cost effectiveness, a key criterion. This was reinforced in the RCM's Vision 2000 (RCM 2000), which emphasized the need to develop a maternity service that provided high-quality, evidence-based, cost-effective care, responsive to individual needs and preferences. Principle number ten in the Vision stated that maternity services should ensure that an evidence base underpins policies and guidelines, and that all staff have access to appropriate education so that they can effectively use research evidence in practice.

However, it is not easy to base practice on research, indeed, research is not readily available on every topic. Even where this form of evidence is available, midwives may not be aware of it, or have easy access to it. They also need to have a sufficient understanding of research to critically assess its quality and value. This is crucial if weak evidence is not to be mistaken for strong, one reason why the Vision placed emphasis on access to education on research.

It is little wonder then, that in many situations other sources of knowledge rather than research influence action. This is not necessarily wrong, however, it is important to recognize that the value put on evidence will vary with its source. In this chapter these alternative forms of knowledge will be examined and contrasted with the use of research-based knowledge.

Sources of midwifery knowledge

What are the sources of knowledge you use in making clinical decisions? Think back to your most recent working day. As you replay it in your mind, list some of the things you did, and identify what has influenced the way you carry out that activity. The result should include some of the following identified by several writers (Cluett and Bluff 2000; Polit et al 2001; Burns and Grove 2001).

♦ *Tradition* (always done it that way)
♦ *Authority/policy* (told to do it that way)
♦ *Education/training* (taught/learnt to do it that way)
♦ *Personal experience* (found it usually works)
♦ *Trial and error* (tried several other ways first)
♦ *Role modelling* (seen others do it this way)
♦ *Intuition* (feels right this way)
♦ *Research* (the research I have read suggest this is the best method).

Some of these will be used more frequently as a source of decision making than others. It may be that research does not figure very prominently on your list. The aim of the exercise is not to make you feel guilty, but to sensitize you to the way in which decisions are influenced by sources of knowledge that will range in their accuracy and effectiveness. The list above consists of two kinds of knowledge; firstly, knowledge relating to *how* to do something, that is, practical skills. The second category relates to knowing *why* we do something, that is, understanding the rationale for activities. In the past, where practice was often influenced by ritual and routine, knowing how to do something was valued in the professional. However, it is just as important to know why we do something so that we can ensure it is the most appropriate choice of action. Research provides one source of knowing why we do something.

Is research really better than the other sources of knowledge? According to Polit et al (2001), research carried out in a disciplined way is the most sophisticated method of acquiring knowledge that humans have developed. The justification for this claim is provided by their description of the scientific approach:

> The traditional scientific approach to inquiry refers to a general set of orderly, disciplined procedures used to acquire information. The traditional scientist uses deductive reasoning to generate hunches that are tested in the real world. In scientific research ... the researcher moves in a systematic fashion from the definition of a problem and the selection of concepts on which to focus, to the solution of the problem. Systematic means that the scientific investigator progresses logically through a series of steps, according to a specified plan of action. The researcher uses, to the extent possible, mechanisms designed to control the study. Control involves imposing conditions on the research situation so that biases are minimized and precision and validity are maximized.
> (p. 13/14)

They go on to suggest that one of the reasons for this systematic and careful approach is so that we can generalize from the findings of a particular study to other situations, and that this ability is one way to assess the quality and importance of a research study.

This provides some clues on the key qualities of research, such as an orderly approach to data collection, knowledge derived from information gathered in the real world (as opposed to simply theorizing) and the use of deductive reasoning. These qualities can now be used to construct a list of the characteristics that differentiate research knowledge from other forms of knowledge (see Box 1.1).

- ◆ An orderly and systematic process of gathering information
- ◆ Control over the process in which the information is gathered
- ◆ Objective evidence of a 'factual nature' taken from real situations (empirical evidence)
- ◆ Absence of individual bias
- ◆ Use of logic in analyzing the information
- ◆ Can be applied to other settings (generalizability).

Box 1.1   Characteristics of research

Taking these in turn we can examine how these alternative sources of knowledge compare with research.

Tradition

One of the big advantages of using tradition as a way of making decisions is that it requires the minimum of thought, and its use is highly acceptable. As tradition suggests a procedure that has been carried out in a set way for some time, it seems likely that there was a good reason for choosing it in the first place. It is also likely that traditional activities are acceptable to those receiving midwifery care, as they are likely to expect a certain procedure or solution to a problem. One description of tradition by Burns and Grove (2001) is that it consists of 'truths' or beliefs that are based on customs and past trends.

It is not difficult to see the weakness of this source of knowledge; it does not necessarily mean that because a practice has been around for a long time that it is beneficial or the best choice. Behi and Nolan (1995) point out that procedures that are accepted simply because of regular and persistent use may have been based on an initial error, and subsequently accepted in an uncritical fashion. From the criteria list in Box 1.1, there is little to support traditional knowledge. Although it is sometimes generalized to other settings and justified on the basis of its acceptance elsewhere, this does not provide sufficient justification for its use.

This basis for decision-making has been the source of many research projects within midwifery. So, for instance, Walsh (2000) has reviewed some of the studies which have looked at the midwife's attempt to control labouring women's urge to push, and the time limits applied to an acceptable length of the second stage of delivery. Interestingly, despite research that suggests women should be allowed to push when it feels right to them, it seems that midwives are reluctant to let go of traditional control of this process.

Authority/policy

The main advantage of basing decisions on policy or the rules and regulations of an authority figure is protection against criticism. It is easy to justify decisions by saying 'I have no choice'. There is also the advantage for the practitioner in knowing where to find an acceptable answer to what should be done. From a service management perspective, if people act in accordance with current policy, then it is possible to achieve a common and consistent approach to activities. It is also a way of achieving control over what might be dubious or poor practices.

The disadvantage is that once policies are accepted they are rarely questioned or challenged, even when circumstances change. They become outdated and difficult to adapt because of the security people feel in following authority. Behi and Nolan (1995) point out that guidelines provided by those in authority may not always be as objective as we may think. Individuals may use their position to ensure that others conform to their personal beliefs or preferences. Accepting without question the word of those in authority, Behi and Nolan suggest, can inhibit the development of an open and questioning approach to professional activities. This is why the production of clinical standards should state the source of knowledge underpinning them, so that standards can change with the development of new knowledge.

Education/training

Education and training as a basis for decision-making is very similar to authority, in that it provides a respected source of knowledge. We are professionally accountable to use only procedures for which we have been trained. It is easy to assume that if we were taught to do things a certain way, then there must have been a sound reason for it.

The disadvantage of this form of knowledge is that it is difficult to move on and develop other ways of making decisions because of the strength of learnt and 'authorized' behaviour. As with policy and authority, education tends to maintain the status quo. People tend to do things the way they were taught, even though the information or technique could have been learnt a very long time ago. We have to remember that knowledge has a shelf life, and there is a danger in following procedures and practices that have long passed their 'sell-by' date.

Personal experience

This source of knowledge comes from being personally involved in an event, situation, or circumstance (Burns and Grove 2001), and appears to support professional experience and individual initiative. We use this method of decision-making in many situations, so it is a familiar strategy to us. However, personal experience does not necessarily guarantee that it is typical or correct. In other words, it lacks a systematic approach and may not be generalized to other situations. Polit et al (2001) also suggest it can be coloured by biases, and so may be unsound.

Trial and error

This alternative seems quite promising as it does accord more with the criteria listed in Box 1.1. It can be described as an orderly and systematic process of collating information, and does collect objective evidence of a 'factual nature' gathered from real situations. There is also the use of logic in analyzing the information. What is perhaps missing is the control over the process as the person carrying out such an activity may not try all the options available and so miss a better alternative. Despite this, as Behi and Nolan (1995) point out, it can be highly regarded:

> Trial and error is a method that is used and often encouraged in nursing as a means of developing practical knowledge and skills. Unfortunately, the learner can assume something to be true on the basis of very few 'trials', often without confirming his/her belief with others. Furthermore, if widely accepted, such trial and error knowledge can soon constitute a new 'tradition'. Moreover, as a patient one would not appreciate, or accept being at the receiving end of such trials and mistakes, even if it may lead to new knowledge.
> (p.141)

This last point raises the question of ethics. Research attempts to safeguard the individual by including protection for those taking part in research, particularly clinical trials. Because of the 'ad hoc' nature of trial and error, the individual is not assured similar protection. On a practical note, Burns and Grove (2001) suggest this method can be very time consuming, as a number of alternatives may have to be tried before one seems appropriate, but more worrying, they also warn there is a risk of implementing actions that are detrimental to individual health.

Role modelling

Role models are those we aspire to and copy, and can be very influential in the way in which we solve particular problems. We might almost subconsciously adopt the solutions, approaches and techniques we have seen others apply. This source of knowledge has the advantage that if others use it, it will have some support. Where the person is a 'role model' because of accepted high standards and appropriate behaviour, this can be very beneficial in raising or maintaining standards. We now have systems of mentoring where role modelling has an approved form. However, like so many of the other alternatives, just because someone uses a certain approach does not make it right. It could be outdated and not really applicable to the situation in which it is used. As with many of the options in the list, it does not mean that it is beyond challenge.

Intuition

Intuition is not something that is characterized by an attempt to logically develop a solution on the basis of given information. It is something that occurs like a sudden flash of inspiration or insight. It may be the result, as Langford (2001) suggests, of a lucky guess. Looking at the list of the characteristics of research in Box 1.1, there is nothing relating to intuition that can be said to compare to research knowledge. It is almost impossible to justify or say on what it is based. This is illustrated by the definition of intuition used by Behi and Nolan (1995) who say it is 'acquiring knowledge without reasoning or inferring'. On this basis, although we may support the value of intuition or sixth sense, it is not something we would expect to be used as the basis of professional decision-making.

The limitations of research

The conclusion we must reach is that research as a basis for decision-making has so many more advantages than all the other alternatives examined. However, there are a number of points we must consider before passing judgement on these other sources of knowledge. Firstly, we must remember that research findings may not be available to answer every midwifery question. Secondly, the research that is available may, for one reason or another, be flawed. Research findings should be challenged before practitioners change their practice. Thirdly, we have to remember that there may be situations where there is no time for the practitioner to consult the appropriate research. Rose and Parker (1994) remind us that applying knowledge to practice is not so cut and dried; it is often carried out in a very uneasy environment where the midwife has very little time to stop and think.

Where we do make decisions on the basis of these alternative sources of knowledge, we must acknowledge their limitations in comparison to research-based evidence. If midwifery is to be taken seriously as a profession, to draw on the words of Walsh and Ford (1989), it must demonstrate that practice is not based purely upon beliefs, but rather that midwifery is a rational, fact-based discipline, more susceptible to change in the face of research findings and new ideas. The following final words are from Mason (1992), who sums up the argument for using research-based knowledge:

> In spite of the limitations, it is inarguably better to base our practice on research evidence rather than tradition: on science rather than ritual. The rigour of the research process generates evidence that forms a more accurate basis for the delivery of care than tradition, and consistency in care giving is more likely to be achieved through research than through habit.
> (p. 37)

Conducting research

In designing a project, the researcher must remember the vital characteristics that make research so highly favoured as a basis for decision-making. The project should follow the orderly and systematic procedures laid down in the research process (see Chapter 3). The researcher should take care to maintain as much of an objective and unbiased approach to data collection as possible. This equally applies to the way in which the results are interpreted. If these principles are followed, and if there is an attempt to collect information from a representative sample of individuals or objects, then the findings are more likely to be applicable to other situations.

In choosing the research topic, and producing a report of the findings, it is worth asking yourself the question 'on what are decisions about this subject based at the moment?' If the answer is tradition, or personal experience, or even intuition, there could be a strong personal and emotional attachment to these current sources of information. This may produce resistance to change in this area, as well as a reluctance to accept the findings of research. There is not overwhelming support for research findings, particularly where they contradict firmly held views, or where their adoption would mean considerable changes in activity, and values. The relevance of this is that the researcher should anticipate the likely areas of resistance to the research from the start, and ensure that the design and implementation of the research takes these into account.

Critiquing research

In examining published research, check the extent to which the researcher illustrates the characteristics found in Box 1.1. Has the research been conducted fairly, with as little bias as possible? We should feel that the information is objective, and the researcher has taken care in its collection and interpretation.

When reading research, some details or statements may raise an emotionally negative response within us, even to the extent that we do not believe the research, or we feel the researcher has 'fiddled' the results. This may be because we are experiencing a threat to our own value system, and the implicit belief in our own intuition or experience. We have already seen that these may not be accurate. In considering research reports, then, we should be aware of our own biases, and try to keep an open mind, even where the findings contradict our own views and experiences.

Key Points

♦ Midwives draw on a number of different sources of knowledge in order to make decisions. Although each of these sources of knowledge has its strengths, research has a number of distinct advantages over other sources of knowledge.

♦ Research is an orderly and systematic process of gathering information where there is control over the process in which the information is gathered. It produces objective evidence of a factual nature taken from real situations (empirical evidence), where there is an absence of individual bias and a use of logic in analyzing the information. Most importantly there is a greater ability to generalize the findings of research to other settings.

♦ As a profession demonstrating evidenced-based practice, midwives have an obligation to seek out and apply the findings of appropriate research. Although research has its limitations, it is still better than basing practice on ritual and tradition.

References

Behi R and Nolan M (1995) Sources of knowledge in nursing. British Journal of Nursing 4(3): 141–159.

Burns N and Grove S (2001) The Practice of Nursing Research: Conduct, Critique, and Utilization (4th edn). Philadelphia: W.B. Saunders.

Cluett E and Bluff R (2000) From practice to research. In: Cluett E and Bluff R (eds) Principles and Practice of Research in Midwifery. Edinburgh: Baillière Tindall.

Langford R (2001) Navigating the Maze of Nursing Research. St. Louis: Mosby.

Mason C (1992) Research in practice: rhetoric or reality? Nursing Standard 6(27): 36–39.

Miller J (2002) Clinical Governance: Nursing Times Clinical Monographs No 56. London: NT Books.

Polit D, Beck C and Hungler B (2001) Essentials of Nursing Research: Methods, Appraisal, and Utilization (5th edn). Philadelphia: Lippincott.

RCM (2000) Vision 2000. London: Royal College of Midwives.

Rose P and Parker D (1994) Nursing: an integration of art and science within the experience of the practitioner. Journal of Advanced Nursing 20(6): 1004–10.

Walsh D (2000) Evidence-Based Care: Part six: Limits on pushing and time in the second stage. British Journal of Midwifery 8(10): 604–608.

Walsh M and Ford P (1989) Nursing Rituals: Research and Rational Action. Oxford: Butterworth-Heinemann.

CHAPTER TWO
Some Important Concepts

Learning about a new topic such as research involves two processes; firstly discovering and understanding unfamiliar words or concepts, and secondly discovering some of the issues related to those concepts. An issue may be defined as a situation where there is a difference of opinion over a topic, such as elective caesarian sections, or a problem that needs a solution, such as increasing the number of breastfeeding mothers.

This chapter will examine some of the important concepts used by researchers. Many midwives may see this as unnecessary jargon, as it often forms a barrier to understanding research. However, in reality, the words form a shorthand for complex concepts, and once the most commonly used words are understood, research can take on a completely different level of understanding. An important starting point is to recognize that research takes in many different forms; in this book we will distinguish midwifery research from that of other disciplines.

Midwifery research

So far we have managed to get to Chapter 2 without defining research. There are a number of dangers in continuing without one. Firstly, we will get to the end of the book and never discover what it was about. Secondly, readers may be forced to use their own definitions of the term, which means different people will have different things in mind. These personal definitions may not be the same as the author intended. We need, then, to give a clear definition of how it is used in this book.

Research can be defined as a process that extends knowledge and understanding through the systematic collection of information that answers a specific question objectively and as accurately as possible. It has similarities to the process of audit, but goes further in the way it increases understanding and is placed within a context of professional knowledge. That is, it is usually placed within the background of previous research that has examined the same topic. Audit is usually interested in the performance of the service, or a part of it, and the comparison of results against an agreed standard (or previous audit results) that may allow action to be taken. Chaffer and Royle (2000) distinguish between the two activities by saying that research is concerned with discovering the right thing to do, whereas audit ascertains whether the right thing has been done.

One of the simplest and frequently quoted definitions of research is that by Macleod Clark and Hockey (1989), cited by Hockey (2000) as follows:

Research is an attempt to increase the sum of what is known, usually referred to as 'a body of knowledge', by the discovery of new facts or relationships through a process of systematic scientific enquiry, the research process.

One problem in trying to define research is that it is similar to words such as 'care', 'delivery', or 'midwifery'; it is used as though it consisted of a single entity when if fact in can take many different forms. And this can lead to confusion. In the above definition, the word 'scientific' is used which may have connotations of people in white coats working in laboratories, when research can be carried out in many settings, and take a variety of forms and sizes. At this stage it is useful to think of research as a process that should conform to a number of principles or guidelines, but these will change depending on the broad nature or category of the research.

Abbott (2002) provides a final definition. Although she is talking about nursing research, it is easy to substitute the word midwifery for nursing. Its inclusion here is to highlight some of the issues in regard to midwifery and research.

Nursing research is the systematic investigation of nursing practice and the effects of this practice on patient care on individual, family or community health. It is new knowledge generated by finding valid answers to questions that have been raised with respect to the care of patients generally or of a particular group of patients/clients. The expectation is that research findings will be generalisable beyond the immediate context.
(p. 15)

This definition brings out the extensive scope of research in midwifery that touches the broad area of hospital, and community care and the wider community health role. It is not simply about individual outcomes, but also caring processes. As with medical research, the systematic way in which it is undertaken means that it should be possible to apply the specific knowledge gained or the broad principles indicated, to situations other than the one in which the study took place.

In order to provide evidence-based practice, the midwife may draw on research carried out by a number of different disciplines. Medical or obstetric research, for instance, will consider a number of clinical issues that will help the midwife both in terms of knowledge and action, and may be useful in helping to empower women to understand when they may have to take action themselves. In the same way, research from psychology or sociology may well provide illuminating information on how people behave and help the midwife in planning care. Research from education and the field of communication may also be relevant. However, the emphasis of this book is on midwifery research. This can be defined as research that describes and explores the problems and issues of direct concern to the midwife and that has implications for the work of the midwife more than any other discipline.

Quantitative and qualitative research

These concepts distinguish two very different approaches to research that are based on contrasting beliefs or philosophies regarding the nature of knowledge. Although the difference between them will be considered in more detail in Chapter 4 on quantitative and qualitative research, it is important that we gain some understanding of the basic differences between them now, and their implication for midwifery research.

Historically, research has been synonymous with the word 'scientific', which is taken to mean objective and accurate. The basic belief on which it is based is that the natural or 'real' world lies outside the experience of the individual and is open to study and quantification. In other words it can be measured in some way. This type of research can be characterized as quantitative as it attempts to quantify elements, such as blood pressure, by means of a numeric value. These numbers can be summarized and may allow the use of a range of statistical techniques. This scientific view or 'paradigm' (model) of research is the one embraced by medical research as the right and proper approach for a profession that concentrates on clinical outcomes. We must remember, however, that this is only one approach to research, and although it is useful in midwifery, there are other, just as legitimate ways of conducting a study besides 'counting' or measuring something.

Qualitative research (sometimes referred to as naturalistic research as it avoids 'controlling' situations) has a different view of the world and the best way of conducting research in it. This approach believes the real world can only be understood through our personal experience of it. Everything depends on how we view it. This explains why some people are afraid of spiders or going to the dentist. It is a product of how people experience them, or the associations they hold for the individual. It does not mean that spiders or dentists themselves are frightening. Naturalistic or qualitative researchers believes that if we are to understand a topic we need to look at it through the eyes of those who experience it, and try to understand it from their point of view. This type of research produces qualitative data in the form of direct quotes, dialogue or extensive descriptions of human activity. It uses such methods as interviews or observations that attempt to capture perceptions, interpretations, experiences or behaviour.

One of the guiding principles of qualitative research is that it attempts to encourage people to express their perceptions of situations or feelings in their own words. So, questionnaires with fixed choice options would not be classed as qualitative research even though they may have tried to see things from the individual's point of view. The reason for this is that the list of alternative answers has been developed by the researcher, and the format does not allow the individual to express answers in their own words, only in those of the researcher.

An important visual distinction between quantitative and qualitative research is the way in which findings are presented. Quantitative research will use graphical forms of data presentation such as tables, bar charts and histograms (more of these in Chapter 13 on statistics). This form of data presentation is not a main feature of qualitative research, although some may present the themes that emerged in a study in the form of a table, showing how many people mentioned each theme (this is known as a frequency table). A qualitative report may also include a table showing details of the sample such as age, number of children, etc. However, it is more usual for qualitative results to avoid numbers and simply present a broad theme heading and discuss the type of comments made, often with examples of quotes or dialogue.

As will be seen in Chapter 4, the differences between these two forms of research are so different they are almost two different entities. The importance of this is that we must avoid criticizing qualitative research using the criteria of a quantitative approach. Which approach is best suited to midwifery? The answer is the one that is most appropriate to the question posed. If the question is one of quantity, or frequency, particularly in regard to clinical outcomes, then a quantitative approach will be appropriate; if the question is one of perceptions, experiences or social processes, then the best approach will be qualitative.

Levels of questions in research

There is no shortage of questions that need to be answered through midwifery research. From the research point of view, it is the question posed by the researcher that acts as the aim of the research. In this book the phrase *terms of reference* will be used to mean the research question. The terms of reference usually begins with the word 'to' as in:

> The aim of this study is **to find out if research evidence was being used in practice [by midwives] and why it would not be used in practice.**
> Richens (2002) p. 11

The section in bold italics would form the terms of reference. This is what the researcher 'refers to' when carrying out the study and gives it direction.

It is important to realize that research questions differ in their complexity and this will have implications for the structure of the study. Brink and Wood (1994) make a useful distinction between what they call the three levels of research question. These levels are influenced by how much is known about a particular subject, or how much theory exists in relation to it.

Level one questions form the most basic level where very little is known about the topic. The purpose of this type of research is to describe a situation. The work of Stewart and Henshaw (2002) is an example of this, where the purpose was to explore the level of knowledge about the prevalence of perinatal mental health disorders (PMHDs) amongst midwives, to ascertain the level of experience they have had in managing women with these problems, and to explore perceptions of their potential role, skill deficits and awareness of a need to improve practice in this area. As can be seen, there are several aspects to this study; each part, however, is a level one question, as there is only one variable being pursued at a time. As there is little known about this situation the purpose of the study is to attempt to gain some basic information on the topic. Stewart and Henshaw (2002) answer these questions in a level one survey and base their results on 266 (70%) responses from midwives who replied to a questionnaire.

Level two questions are those where some basic information is known about a topic, and there is an attempt to look for a possible relationship between two or more factors. The work of Mead et al (2000) is one such study that compared intrapartum care in four neighbouring maternity units. The rates of normal instrumental deliveries and caesarean sections were compared in association with the use of augmentation of labour, electronic fetal monitoring and epidural analgesia. The results based on 4203 cases indicated a higher rate of intervention was associated with higher rates of instrumental deliveries and caesarian sections. They emphasize that the single most important factor associated with a rise in the caesarian section rate was the use of epidural analgesia. The authors use the data to suggest that levels of intervention may be driven more by policy and procedure than by the biological needs of women.

Level three questions are used to test hypotheses based on already established theories about a topic. The work by Steen and Marchant (2001) would be an example of this. Their randomized control trial evaluated the effectiveness of a new cooling device (gel pad) in comparison with a standard regimen (ice pack) and no localized treatment regimen (control). The study drew on theory concerning the reduction of pain, oedema and bruising through the use of cooling agents. The trial, which involved 316 women, demonstrated that a specifically designed cooling gel pad is a safe and effective localized method to alleviate perineal trauma without any adverse effects on healing.

These three levels form an important distinction, as they influence the type of approach the researcher must use to gather the data. Level one questions require a descriptive approach using perhaps survey methods or a qualitative approach. Level two questions require more sophistication in the method of analysis in order to suggest that relationships between variables may exist. Finally, level three questions require the use of an experimental approach that will test whether a hypothesis based on a theory can be supported by research evidence. Each level also requires more from those making use of the research as the amount of research knowledge and critical analysis increases in complexity with each level.

Variables

At this point we can examine some of the concepts that form the basic building blocks of research. Once we are familiar with their meaning we should find a difference in our ability to analyze research.

All studies are concerned with examining specified elements of interest to the researcher, such as pain in delivery, breastfeeding problems, professional updating and so on. The term 'variable' is used to describe these items as they differ or vary in some way. For example, length of labour, attitude towards natural childbirth methods, social class, temperature, and level of pain in labour, can vary from one person to another. Burns and Grove (2001:182) state that *'variables are qualities, properties, or characteristics of persons, things, or situations that change or vary and are manipulated, measured or controlled in research'*. We should, therefore, attempt to identify the particular variables of concern in the studies we examine.

In level three questions involving randomized control trials we can often subdivide variables into two types: *dependent variables* and *independent variables*. The variable that is the focus of concern to the researcher is the dependent variable, such as continuity of care, or level of pain. The variable that is presumed to play a part in influencing the dependent variable is known as the independent variable. An example will make this clear. Imagine that a researcher wishes to examine whether women who have attended antenatal classes feel more involved with their delivery than those who have not attended classes. The extent to which women feel involved with their delivery would be the dependent variable; attendance at antenatal classes would be the independent variable. The independent variable can be thought of as the influencing factor or 'cause' and the dependent factor is the outcome consequence, or 'effect'. Experimental research, which we shall explore later in Chapter 12, revolves around the examination of cause and effect relationships, where the researcher introduces the independent variable into the experimental group and examines its effect on outcomes.

Initially, the difference between dependent and independent variables can be difficult to grasp. An easy way of sorting them out is to think of their chronological order, and identify which comes first and which comes last. The variable that comes first in time is the independent variable – the influence, and the variable that comes last is the dependent variable – the outcome. In the example above, attendance at antenatal classes happens before feelings of involvement in delivery, so attendance would be the independent variable, and the feeling of control, the dependent variable.

One danger in studies like this is that they appear to be based on the assumption that events are influenced by only one factor. Things are rarely as simple as this, and a number of other variables may influence whether a woman feels involved with their delivery. Other factors such as personality, the quality of the relationship with their birth partner, parity and social class may all play a part. These would also be independent variables that the researcher may need to consider. In any study, then, we should identify the dependent variable and the independent variable. We should then ask, 'is there anything else that could have influenced the outcome that has not been taken into account?' If we do this, then we are becoming a more critical user of research.

Concept definitions and operational definitions

These two concepts explain what the researcher means by the words used to describe the study variables, and how they were measured. The *concept definition* is a clear statement of the sense in which the researcher is using the words describing the concept. It is similar in some ways to a dictionary definition of the word. In our example of attendance at antenatal classes and feelings of involvement, although we may feel we do not need the words 'antenatal classes' defined, there are a variety of terms used to describe them in the UK, and they may well not mean the same to readers from other countries. We would also be concerned about the concept definition of what qualifies as 'attendance at classes'. If someone attended just one or two sessions are they referred to as having attended in the same way as those who have attended six or eight? The other term we would want clearly defined would be 'feelings of involvement'. What exactly does this mean? To provide an answer, criteria may be provided that specifies what counts as feelings of involvement. These might include whether options for intervention were discussed, whether the final decision was left to the individual, and whether questions and queries were fully answered and so on.

The meaning of the term *operational definition* is important from the data-gathering point of view, as it indicates how a particular concept is to be measured or 'operationalized'. Polit et al (2001:34) define the operational definition as *'the specification of the operations that the researcher must perform to collect the required information'*. So, for instance, condition of the baby following birth may be operationalized using the Apgar score that will permit different babies to be compared following delivery. Concepts such as pain are more difficult, but now pain scores may be used to operationalize levels of pain. In a study of health problems following delivery, Bick and MacArthur (1995) asked women to mark on a 100 mm line how severe their symptoms had been for health problems they had experienced. This calibrated line is known as a visual analogue scale (VAS) and is used in a number of studies to operationalize concepts that do not usually have a numeric value attached to them. The line is divided into 25 mm sections so that the location of a cross, indicated by a respondent along the line can be given a numeric value, and comparisons made between respondents.

Theoretical and conceptual frameworks

One of the aims of research is to add to the body of knowledge on a particular subject, and to increase understanding by developing a more accurate theory about why things happen the way they do.

A particular study cannot look at everything and will confine itself to a number of key factors or variables. The researcher's understanding of those variables can be expressed in terms of the theoretical framework that is adopted for the study. This provides a clear context for the study. Burns and Grove (2001:141) define a theory as *'an integrated set of defined concepts and existence statements, and relational statements that present a view of a phenomenon and can be used to describe, explain, predict and/or control that phenomenon.'*

Bryar (1995), who is one of the few writers on midwifery theory, suggests that theory sensitizes midwives to the things that they should be watching for and helps to identify those factors that are central to care from those factors that are less important.

Theories can be categorized in several ways such as formal, informal or personal theories. An example of a formal theory would be Rotter's theory on internal and external locus of control. This psychological theory suggests that people differ in the extent to which they believe they can influence their own destinies and the things that happen to them. Those with an internal locus of control believe that they can influence to a large extent what happens to them. Those with an external locus believe that no matter how hard they try, it is those with greater power than themselves, organizations or even fate that dictate their destiny. The application of this theory to midwifery research would be to examine whether attendance at antenatal classes is influenced by an individual's locus of control. From this, a hypothesis could be constructed that those with an internal locus of control are more likely to attend because they will feel they can influence what happens to them throughout pregnancy and childbirth once they have the relevant knowledge.

Personal or informal theories are those beliefs we hold, frequently at a subconscious level, which influence our behaviour. We may encourage women to construct a birth plan because we believe that women are more likely to voice their own opinion if they have first thought about them, and then committed them to paper. The midwifery researcher may use a formal theory, or personal theory as the basis of a study.

American nursing theorists have influenced nursing research to some extent, and studies have concentrated on such elements as adaptation, self-care and stressors, as outlined in various nursing theories. However, it can be argued that as midwifery has different concerns and relationships with those with whom they are in contact, midwifery research should draw on midwifery concepts and theories. However, as Bryar (1995) points out, this is no easy matter, as midwifery does not seem to have developed its ideas as systematically as nursing. Although Bryar does present five midwifery theorists on whom it may be possible to develop midwifery research, four of these are American nurse-midwives, and only one, Jean Ball, is a British midwife. Interestingly, the key concepts of 'Changing Childbirth' (DoH, 1993), namely 'choice', 'control' and 'continuity', are still used in midwifery research as an organizing framework.

The relationship between concepts is sometimes presented diagrammatically to illustrate how the author visualizes the links between the dependent and independent variable(s). These diagrams are sometimes referred to as conceptual frameworks or conceptual maps, where key concepts are joined by lines and arrows to show the direction and nature of the relationships believed to exist. So a study may concentrate on the concept of breastfeeding, and be concerned with some of the independent variables, which may influence the adoption of breastfeeding. A suitable conceptual framework that would illustrate the researcher's thinking may look something like Figure 2.1.

As can be seen, conceptual frameworks provide a mental image of what the researcher sees as the influencing factors or variables that will be explored in a study. This provides the researcher with a clear picture of the topic areas that should be included in the tool of data collection.

Conceptual frameworks can also develop as a result of data gathering, particularly in qualitative research. So Levy (1999) developed a conceptual framework in her grounded theory study of the way in which midwives facilitate informed choices during pregnancy, and presented this schematically.

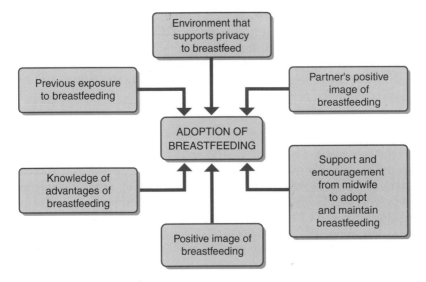

Fig. 2.1 Conceptual framework for a study exploring the decision to breastfeed

Polit et al (2002) point out that not all research is linked to a conceptual framework. This is particularly true where the study is very pragmatic, that is, based on practical outcomes. Where a study does draw on one, the design of the study, the key concepts, and the analyzes and interpretation of data should all flow from that conceptualization. In other words, they are a very powerful part of a research process. It is for this reason that a thorough review of the literature is essential to provide the theoretical and conceptual context for the study. This will then provide a clear indication of the key concepts to be selected, and possible concept and operational definitions.

One final word is to emphasize that the use of theories and conceptual frameworks do vary between quantitative research, which will usually start with a theory and conceptual framework, and qualitative research, which is more likely to develop one during or following data analysis. Remember, not all studies will make use of theoretical and conceptual frameworks, and they are not a feature of audit.

Reliability, validity, bias and rigour

These concepts may be familiar but their exact meaning may be unclear. Their use relates to quantitative research approaches and is concerned with the nature of measurement.

Reliability

This relates to the method that is being used to collect the data and refers to the accuracy and consistency of the measurements generated by this method. If we wanted to carpet a room, the use of a metre length of elastic to measure the area would make us distrust the reliability of the method of collecting the measurements. Reliability then, is to do with the consistency of the measurement tool. If a study is concerned with weighing a number of babies, we would want to ensure any weighing scales used were first tested for accuracy. Where a number of different scales were used we would want to ensure that each one gave an accurate reading, otherwise the reliability of the results would be open to question.

Validity

This relates to what is being measured and is an attempt to ensure that the research tool is really measuring what the researcher believes it is measuring. So, for instance, we could think we were looking at the satisfaction of women with the clinical skills of their midwife, when we were really measuring the influence of the midwife's personality that may influence how women felt about the care they received. Although reliability is usually amenable to checking, and may become apparent in a pilot study, validity is far more difficult to confirm.

Bias

The degree of accuracy in the results of a study will be influenced by the amount of *bias* contained in the research. Bias has been defined by Polit et al (2001) as any influence that produces a distortion in the results of a study. This can take a number of different forms, as we shall see in later sections. Here, we will concentrate on bias within the sample that may make them untypical or unrepresentative of the group they represent (see Chapter 14). This can happen through the method of selection.

In describing the sample the researcher frequently mentions the inclusion and exclusion criteria used to select those in the study. These terms relate to the characteristics of those felt to be typical of the study group – the *inclusion criteria*, and those characteristics that were felt may either put them at clinical risk, or that would introduce bias into the group – the *exclusion criteria*. It is important to examine these closely and assess whether you feel the researcher has attempted to control for bias in the way the sample was selected. Look out too for any changes in the size of the groups as a result of people dropping out of a study. This may make it difficult to carry on comparing groups, as they may no longer be similar in composition once a number of people have dropped out of the study.

Rigour

This concept relates to the overall planning and implementation of the research design. It addresses the issue of whether the researcher has carried out the study in a logical, systematic way and paid attention to factors that may influence the accuracy of the results. Burns and Grove (2001) suggest that rigour is the *striving for excellence* in research and involves discipline, adherence to detail, and strict accuracy. They argue that a rigorously conducted study has precise measurement tools, a representative sample, and a tightly controlled study design. They also make the point that rigour applies just as much to qualitative research as quantitative, where poorly developed methods, inadequate time spent gathering and analyzing the data can all put the quality of the research at risk. LoBiondo-Wood and Haber (2002) also support the view that the qualitative researcher is just as concerned with the soundness of their data, although they will employ different methods to ensure the accuracy and generalizability of their results, as we shall see in Chapter 4.

Midwifery is a discipline that needs to draw on both quantitative and qualitative research approaches. The issues and problems with which it is concerned relate to both the worlds of quantification found in the scientific approach, and the naturalistic world as experienced by those who come into contact with midwifery services, including midwives themselves. This book will concern itself with this wide spectrum of research approaches and illustrate how they have been applied to the concerns of midwives.

Conducting research

The key research concepts included in this chapter form the basic thought processes used by the researcher at the planning stage of a project. Understanding them is vital. It is like having a basic vocabulary in a foreign language that will allow you to cope with most of the situations you are likely to encounter.

The distinction between quantitative and qualitative research involves two contrasting broad approaches to research. In quantitative research, the researcher will design a study that collects information in numeric form that may be summarized and manipulated statistically. Qualitative research, on the other hand, will mean the researcher will collect data, mainly in the form of words, either as the result of interviews, or observations. The approach used will depend very much on the nature of the research question, and what kind of data is implicitly implied in the terms of reference.

Similarly, the researcher must have knowledge of the three levels of research questions in order to design the study at the right level. The level is based on the amount of knowledge already available on that topic and the purpose of the study. This means before the researcher can be specific about the level of the research question they must carry out a comprehensive review of the literature to establish the appropriate level of question required in the study.

The review of the literature should also help the researcher define the variables and provide a concept and operational definition for each one. Where the study is level two or three, the researcher should identify which is the dependent and which is the independent variable(s).

Critiquing research

Research articles can seem to be written in a foreign language unless the reader has a basic understanding of the concepts introduced in this chapter. Once these have been mastered the reader will not only understand far more, but will become more appreciative of good research, and will become more critical of weak research.

Knowing the distinction between quantitative and qualitative research will help anticipate the appropriate research approach, and the type of data collected. As will be seen in Chapter 5, there are two different approaches to critiquing an article depending on whether it is quantitative or qualitative in design.

An ability to identify the level of the research question will allow the reader to make certain assumptions about the research and the form it will take. Knowing the levels also provides a way of critically examining the study to ensure that the researcher has conformed to the implications of the different levels, and has not carried out something that is inappropriate to that level.

In reading a research report, a reader should quickly establish the variables under scrutiny. The clarity of the concept and operational definitions will ensure the reader knows exactly what the researcher is looking at, and how it is being measured. Where the question is level three, the reader should identify which are the dependent and independent variables in order to follow what is going on.

The underlying theoretical or conceptual framework will also allow the reader to understand why the particular elements have been linked and the underlying assumptions that have been made by the researcher. In identifying the theoretical or conceptual framework, the reader should ensure that the items in the tool of data collection, and the discussion of the findings reflect the framework. At the moment, very little midwifery research makes the theoretical or conceptual framework to a study explicit.

Critiquing is about assessing how well the researcher has accomplished the design and presentation of their research. It is an assessment of both the strengths and weakness of a written or verbal research presentation. In order to provide a fair assessment, the reader must always keep the concepts of reliability, validity, bias and rigour in mind. These concepts provide an informed approach to assessing firstly, the quality of the research, and secondly, the degree of excellence achieved by the researcher.

Key Points

◆ Research depends on an understanding of some key concepts relating to how the researcher defines the topic(s) of interest.

◆ Quantitative and qualitative methods relate to the different approaches to research design, and are based on philosophical beliefs about the nature of empirical evidence. Quantitative research is based on the belief that information lies outside the personal views of the individual. It emphasizes accuracy, and produces numerical data. Qualitative researchers believe that knowledge is produced by our subjective experience, and that we need to look at things from our respondent's point of view. Midwifery is concerned with issues that draw on both approaches.

◆ Research questions can relate to three levels of exploration. Level one questions relate to describing one variable, usually about which little is known, or that has rarely been the subject of research. Level two questions look for relationships between variables but where little theory exists. Level three questions relate to questions where theory exists and the aim is to test hypotheses based on the theory.

◆ Variables are the elements in which the researcher is interested. In level three questions, there will usually be a dependent variable that is the outcome or effect, and one or more independent variables that are presumed to influence or cause the dependent variable.

◆ Concept definitions relate to how the researcher defines the topic in which they are interested. This can be thought of as a dictionary definition or alternative word for the topic of interest.

◆ Operational definitions refer to the way in which a concept is measured. It reduces the vagueness of such words as comfort, satisfaction, and benefit, by producing a clear specification of how the researcher will make them visible in a specific study.

◆ Theoretical and conceptual frameworks provide the context and meaning for the ideas and concepts contained in a study.

◆ Reliability, validity, bias and rigour relate to firstly, the extent to which the tool of data collection is accurate and consistent between different measurements, or different researchers. Validity relates to whether the method does measure what the researcher intends it to measure. Bias is the extent to which the findings are distorted either by the choice of subjects or the method of measurement. Rigour is the extent to which the researcher has attempted to conduct the study to ensure accuracy and a high quality piece of work.

References

Abbott P (2002) Implementing evidence-informed nursing: research awareness. In: McSherry R, Simmonds M and Abbot P (eds) Evidence-Informed Nursing: A Guide for Clinical Nurses. London: Routledge.

Bick D and MacArthur C (1995) The extent, severity and effect of health problems after childbirth. British Journal of Midwifery 3(1): 27–31.

Brink P and Wood M (1994) Basic Steps in Planning Nursing Research (4th edn). Boston: Jones and Bartlett.

Bryar R (1995) Theory for Midwifery Practice. Houndmills: Macmillan.

Burns N and Grove S (2001) The Practice of Nursing Research: Conduct, Critique, and Utilization (4th edn). Philadelphia: W.B. Saunders.

Chaffer D and Royle L (2000) The use of audit to explain the rise in caesarean section. British Journal of Midwifery 8(11): 677–684.

Department of Health (1993) Changing Childbirth. The Report of the Expert Maternity Group. London: HMSO.

Hockey L (2000) The nature and purpose of research. In: Cormack D (ed) The Research Process in Nursing (4th edn). Oxford: Blackwell Scientific.

Levy V (1999) Protective steering: a grounded theory study of the processes by which midwives facilitate informed choices during pregnancy. Journal of Advanced Nursing 29(1): 104–112.

LoBiondo-Wood G and Haber J (2002) Nursing Research: Methods, Critical Appraisal, and Utilization (5th edn). St. Louis: Mosby.

Mead M, O'Connor R and Kornbrot D (2000) A comparison of intrapartum care in four maternity units. British Journal of Midwifery 8(11): 709–715.

Polit D, Beck B and Hungler B (2001) Essentials of Nursing Research: Methods, Appraisal, and Utilization (5th edn). Philadelphia: Lippincott.

Richens Y (2002) Are midwives using research evidence in practice? British Journal of Midwifery 10(1): 11–16.

Steen M and Marchant P (2001) Alleviating perineal trauma – the APT study. RCM Midwives Journal 4(8): 256–259.

Stewart C and Henshaw C (2002) Midwives and perinatal mental health. British Journal of Midwifery 10(2): 117–121.

CHAPTER THREE
The Basic Framework of Research

An understanding of the basic framework of research projects is imperative, whether you are intending to carry out research or read research articles. This chapter will outline the stages involved in designing and carrying out a research project. The framework used here applies fundamentally to quantitative research projects. Although qualitative research follows similar steps, the order of the stages may be different. The next chapter will provide more detail on the distinction between these two approaches.

What is involved in carrying out research? There are two ways this can be examined; firstly by identifying the broad phases of a project, and secondly by looking at the more detailed stages contained within the phases. Polit et al (2001) have outlined the main phases of quantitative research as follows:

◆ *The Conceptual Phase*   This is the main thinking phase where the researcher develops the idea for the research, and gradually develops a researchable question.

◆ *The Design and Planning Phase*   This includes decisions on the broad research approach and the tool of data collection.

◆ *The Empirical Phase*   This involves collecting information and includes the pilot study, which tests the method.

◆ *The Analytic Phase*   In this part the data are analyzed and a report written.

◆ *The Dissemination Phase*   Finally, the research report is communicated to those who can best benefit from it. The final section of the report or article should include the recommendations for how the findings can be utilized, so that practice can benefit.

This outline demonstrates that research consists of a sandwich of:

THINKING – DOING – THINKING.

The attributes of a researcher should therefore include an emphasis on analytical ability. Parahoo (1997) also highlights the role of the researcher's beliefs and values in influencing the way the research will be carried out. So although we may concentrate on the processes the researcher follows from beginning to end we should not lose sight of the thinking behind them that will influence their nature.

We can now look at the broad phases outlined above in terms of the stages within them. The overall structure of the research process is summarized in Box 3.1.

1. Develop the research question.
2. Review the relevant literature.
3. Plan the method of investigation.
   This includes:
   a) The broad approach i.e. quantitative or qualitative
   b) The sample, sample size, and sampling strategy
   c) The information to be gathered
   d) The tool of data collection
   e) The form of data analysis and presentation
   f) The ethical issues to be addressed before the study is commenced.
4. Carry out a pilot study.
5. Collect the data.
6. Analyze the results.
7. Develop conclusions and recommendations.
8. Communicate the study.

Box 3.1   Stages in the research process

Stage one: The research question

Research begins when the researcher decides to carry out a study on a particular topic. Where do ideas for research come from? Perhaps one of the most common sources is the existence of a problem in the practice area. The researcher's first task is to take the problem and design the research question, or *'terms of reference'*. This is a clear statement of the aim of the project. At the preliminary stage the researcher may think in terms of a question that begins with 'why?' 'what?' 'when?' or 'how?' Brink and Wood (1994) call these words the stem of the question and what comes after them, the topic. An example would be 'what are the factors that influence women to give up breastfeeding?' or 'what attracts certain women to attend antenatal classes and not others?' Giving up breastfeeding, and attraction to antenatal classes would be the topics and 'why' and 'what' would be the stem.

These questions are then converted into terms of reference by removing the stem and replacing it with 'to identify', 'to compare', 'to determine' or a similar phrase that outlines the aim of the study. So for instance, we could say the aim of our study was 'to identify the factors that influence women to give up breastfeeding', or 'to compare the characteristics of women who attend antenatal classes with those who do not'. Table 3.1 illustrates questions that have been developed into terms of reference.

In experimental and some correlation studies, the researcher will usually state a hypothesis, or even more than one. A hypothesis can be defined as a prediction about the relationship between two or more variables (LoBiondo-Wood and Haber 2002). In more simple terms, it is the 'hunch' that the researcher has about the outcome of the study. In experimental studies, the aim is to predict the nature of the relationship between the independent and dependent variables.

Table 3.1   Examples of terms of reference

Author	Question	Terms of reference
Moffat et al (2001)	Is perineal pain following delivery managed better through self or staff administration of paracetamol?	To assess the effect of two different methods of paracetamol administration on perineal pain management.
Ingram et al (2002)	Why do some babies produce excess mucus soon after delivery?	To explore some of the common mediating factors associated with this [excess production of mucus] condition.
Singh et al (2002)	What are the information needs of first-time mothers?	To find out how much information [pregnant] women felt they needed and what topics they wanted to know more about.

Although a hypothesis is not required in descriptive research as the purpose is not to test the relationship between variables, it is sometimes helpful for the researcher to consider what assumptions they hold about influencing factors. These can be used in deciding what information to gather. So in describing what attracts some women to antenatal classes and not others, the researcher might hypothesise that factors such as social class, age and parity may be influential. These would then be included as questions in the tool of data collection.

An important consideration at this stage is whether the question is researchable. Not all questions are amenable to investigation. Philosophical questions, or ethical issues, cannot be answered through research. Such questions as 'should midwives wear a uniform?' or 'should midwives reserve the right to strike?' belong in this category and are really the subject of debate not research.

It must also be possible and practical to answer the research question. This relates to the feasibility of the research and concerns the availability of resources and expertise required to complete the study. Practical elements should always be considered when studies are being planned. Some of these have been highlighted by LoBiondo-Wood and Haber (2002) who make the following observation:

> *The feasibility of a research problem must be pragmatically examined. Regardless of how significant or researchable a problem may be, pragmatic considerations such as time; availability of subjects, facilities, equipment, and money; experience of the researcher; and any ethical considerations may cause the researcher to decide that the problem is inappropriate because it lacks feasibility.* (p. 56)

One of the most important criteria is its relevance to practice. Cluett and Bluff (2000) suggest that the one overriding purpose of research must be to improve the outcomes and experiences of childbirth for all involved in the process. They go on to make the following suggestions for interrelated aims that should be achieved by research to expand midwifery knowledge:

◆   To gain an ever-deepening understanding of the physiological, psychological and sociological aspects of the childbearing process
◆   To develop a sound rationale for midwifery practice
◆   To increase the variety of options available to those involved in the childbearing process
◆   To develop standards of care and thus contribute to quality assurance
◆   To contribute to the provision of cost-effective care.
     (p. 5)

The first stage of research is complex. The type and nature of the question are all important, not only from the professional point of view, but also in relation to the research method. Many of the other stages in the research process will be influenced by the nature of the terms of reference. So, for instance the broad approach, the method of data collection, the sample and method of data analysis can all be implicitly influenced by the aim of the study.

Stage two: reviewing the literature

Studies should not be undertaken in isolation from previous research, therefore the second stage of the research process consists of a critical review of the literature. The aim of this is to gain more information about the topic being examined, and clarify the research question (see Chapter 7). Although this stage is an essential element in quantitative research, in qualitative research the literature is not always consulted at this point; instead it is used at the analysis stage to help make sense of the data gathered. Qualitative researchers avoid examining the literature too early in case their own views are influenced by what they read, and so restrict the topics and issues included in data collection.

In quantitative research, reviewing the literature is an important part of clarifying one's ideas, and a necessary early stage in the research process. Midwifery is extremely fortunate in having such resources as the MIDIRS information system and the Cochrane database to access information on published research. Local midwifery and nursing libraries, especially those with a CD ROM and Internet access, are also part of the process of gathering information on previous studies.

The review is important not only to provide information on the topic, but also to provide guidance on the approach and methods used by those who have studied a particular topic. The 'methods' section of research articles provides useful guidance on the way data can be gathered. Most authors also provide some details of problems encountered and comment on what they would have done differently with hindsight. All these are valuable to the researcher planning a study. Once this stage is reached, Bray and Rees (1995) suggest that the researcher stops, and asks the following three qu

◆ Does it need to be done, or should we be basing practice on the research already available?

◆ What use will be made of the results? It is rarely worth putting a lot of energy into a project where there is little chance of it being implemented.

◆ Can I do it? Do I have the resources, skills and time for this to be carried out rigorously?

Unless the answers to these questions are positive, there may be little point in moving on to the next stage of planning the study.

Stage three: planning the study

Once the first two stages are complete, the researcher is ready to plan the study from beginning to end. The quality of the research will be influenced by the amount of preparation and planning that has been invested in it. Rigour is an important aspect in research, and is dependent on this thinking phase. Box 3.1 lists the considerations that should be included in this planning stage as follows:

The broad research design

This is the blueprint the researcher will follow and is influenced by the purpose of the research. If the researcher aims to establish cause and effect relationships, as in a level three question (see Chapter 2), then the broad approach would be experimental. If the purpose were to describe a situation, as in a level one question, then a descriptive approach would be appropriate using perhaps a survey method. A survey may also be used where the researcher wants to identify if certain variables are related, as in a level two question that looks at correlation.

There are other approaches, such as action research, which is concerned with the introduction of change into the work environment and then evaluating its success and acceptability. This has not become a widely used method in midwifery, and there are few clear examples of its use (Fraser 2000), despite the view that it is approaching a state of maturity in its use in health and social care (le May and Lathlean 2001). The emphasis of action research on change makes it appealing to those who want to move practice forward. It is designed to include those working in the areas affected by a change, and avoids change for its own sake, ensuring that there are benefits over the status quo. To be truly a research approach, however, le May and Lathlean (2001) argue that it should contribute to increasing our understanding or have the potential to be 'theory-generating'. An example of its use would be the introduction and evaluation of a system of patient held notes that looked at women's perception of being responsible for recorded information about themselves.

r method that has not been used a great deal in ial for providing a sense of development within use of historical records and accounts, such as f a particular issue or problem. The work of e where documents, reports and government apervision have been examined to analyze the loped.

ed as a broad research approach. Although not be of audit in midwifery has become so common that it merits reference. Audit requires the same systematic approach and rigour found in research. However, its purpose is not to add to midwifery knowledge, nor can the results of one audit be applied elsewhere, yet it does answer important questions that are very similar to level one research questions.

The sample

The sample relates to the people, items, or events included in the research (see Chapter 14). In the planning stage the researcher must consider the characteristics that make individuals eligible for selection, and those that would make them unsuitable or even put them at risk or at a disadvantage. These considerations form the inclusion and exclusion criteria of a study. The researcher should also attempt to estimate the intended size of the sample. Comparisons with previous research may provide some clue as to optimum size, as well as helping with the sampling method.

Deciding on the data to be collected

In any study it is tempting to collect information simply for the sake of it, out of a belief that everything is relevant and should be included. This will result in information overload and make it difficult to do anything with the findings. The researcher should consider each item to be included and ask two questions:

◆ Is this relevant to my terms of reference?
◆ What use am I going to make of this information?

Unless both of these can be clearly answered the information should not be included.

The method of data collection

There are a number of alternative tools of data collection that can be used to gather information. Those most frequently used include:

◆ Questionnaires
◆ Interviews
◆ Observation
◆ Documentary methods
◆ Experimental methods.

Each one will have its advantages and disadvantages, so how does a researcher know which one to choose? One of the main considerations in selecting the data collection tool is the terms of reference. If the research question is related to staff or women's experiences, views and opinions, and they are in the best position to provide an answer, then questionnaires or interviews will be appropriate. Where the researcher is interested in behaviour or technique, such as methods of conducting antenatal classes, then observation will be a more reliable method. This is true of any question where we are concerned with what people do, rather than with what people say they do. Remember too, that much of our behaviour and actions are so automatic and carried out at a subconscious level, that we may find it difficult to accurately describe what we do. For everyday quantitative data, midwifery notes or the medical record may be the best source of information. Finally, where we are carrying out a level three study where we want to examine the existence of cause and effect relationships, we would use experimental methods, including physiological measurements.

It is possible to use more than one method in a single study and this is called *triangulation*. This is used to overcome the limitations of a single method of collecting data and so increase the validity of the results. As part of triangulation, researchers might interview midwives on how they discuss smoking in pregnancy with mothers, and then observe interactions to provide a fuller picture of what goes on.

The method of analysis and presentation

Whichever method is selected to gather the data, the method of analysis should be considered at the design stage. If the analysis will involve the use of statistics, then the researcher must decide which statistical techniques would be most appropriate (see Chapter 13), or consult someone who can provide advice. At this stage it is also important to think how the results will be presented, especially if one item of information is to be cross-tabulated with another. An example would be where the method of infant feeding is to be presented by parity. The method of analysis will also influence the form in which the information is collected. If the researcher wanted to provide an analysis of the average length of time babies were breastfed, it would be necessary to ask women for the time in weeks and not ask them to tick a box that related to a spread of weeks, for example 3–6 or 7–10 weeks, as averages are calculated on individual figures and not a range.

Ethical issues

Just as the midwife is bound by a professional code of conduct, so the researcher is bound by an ethical code in conducting research. Ethics in research relate to a number of issues that include the following:

- Informed consent
- Confidentiality
- The avoidance of harm or exposure to risk

◆   The avoidance of raising expectations that it may not be possible to meet
◆   The use of a research ethics committee (REC) to approve the study.

All of these issues are covered in more detail in Chapter 8. At the planning stage the researcher must consider the implications of the study for each of these issues and ensure they are addressed when carrying out the study.

Once the planning is complete the researcher may produce a research proposal. This is a written outline of the study and includes the justification for the study, the terms of reference and many of the details developed in the planning phase. The research proposal may be used to gain permission to undertake the study, gain funding or submitted to the ethics committee, if appropriate, to gain ethical approval or to a scientific scrutiny panel to consider the methods being proposed. The importance of gaining this kind of permission and support means that great care and attention should be taken in producing it. The researcher must ensure that they have fully illustrated their ability to complete a worthwhile study (Bond 2000). The production of a proposal is also invaluable to the researcher as it allows them to assess their ideas on paper. This may reveal some problematic aspects of the study that had not been previously apparent.

Stage four: pilot

Before the study is carried out, the researcher must ensure that there are no unanticipated problems in gaining access to the data, and that the method used to collect the data will work. This is the role of the pilot study. Polit et al (2001) define the pilot as a small-scale version, or trial run, carried out in preparation for a major study. Although its purpose usually relates to checking the accuracy of the data collection tool, it should be used to consider a range of factors. These include the whole feasibility in terms of the resources, time, availability of subjects for the study, their willingness to participate and the support required from others to facilitate data collection. All these need to be assessed before a total and perhaps expensive commitment to the study is made.

The results gathered in the pilot should also be analyzed to test the way they will be processed in the main study. The major outcome of the pilot will be the assessment of the reliability of the data collection tool and the opportunity to practise using it. Refinements can then be made that will allow the main study to progress as efficiently as possible. In this way the pilot study is very much like a dress rehearsal that allows all the elements in the study to be tested and adjustments made before the opening night.

Stage five: data collection

Once the pilot had been completed the researcher is in a position to start data collection. As can be seen, this comes quite some way into the total process. Bray and Rees (1995) warn that although the researcher tries to anticipate problems, unexpected things do go wrong. Postal strikes happen once questionnaires have been sent out and delay their return; sickness and absence reduce the number of staff available for interview; and newspapers and tele-vision influence respondents by suddenly promoting the very topic being examined in the study. All this is inevitable and a normal part of the research process.

Stage six: data analysis

Data analysis takes place when the data have been collected. This consists of counting, classifying, and grouping the individual pieces of data so that a broad pattern may be discernible. Descriptive statistics may be used to pre-sent a picture of the results using techniques such as averages (Clegg 1982). Tables and graphs are used to show the results in a visually informative way. Statistical tests or correlation may be used to establish if there are any statis-tical associations present (Clegg 1982). In qualitative research the vast amount of information collected is analyzed to establish themes and categories. These are then compared with the literature to achieve greater validity of the findings, and to help in theory construction.

Stage seven: conclusions and recommendations

The data analysis should lead to conclusions. These should be based on and supported by the results. The conclusion should also provide an answer to the terms of reference, and, where appropriate, say whether the study hypothesis has been accepted or rejected (we do not say proved or disproved because there is always a margin of error). The implications of the findings are then discussed and will result in recommendations both for further research and for changes in practice where appropriate.

Stage eight: communication of findings

Research will only be useful if it is communicated. The last stage in the research process consists of the production of a report, article or verbal presentation where the author will provide the following details:

- What they set out to do
- Why they did it
- How they did it
- What they found
- What it all means.

We can now use this knowledge of the research process in Chapter 5, which covers critiquing research articles and reports. Further chapters will look at some of the topics and issues covered in this chapter in more detail.

Conducting research

This chapter has presented the basic framework the researcher follows in car-rying out research. It is very methodical and has an internal consistency where every stage has implications for further stages. Although it is presented here as a series of steps, it should be acknowledged that some of these are carried out in parallel, or the researcher may go back to certain stages and carry out further work on them. It is not necessarily as neat as it appears.

The essence of good research is planning, and the researcher will increase their chances of a successful project the more time they spend on this stage. The importance of the review of the literature as a source of information and ideas on the research approach should also be emphasized. Above all, the researcher should not be tempted to cut corners by neglecting a pilot study, as so many unanticipated problems can be revealed at this stage.

The feasibility of the study should be carefully considered, and two important elements at the planning stage are firstly to think about permission to conduct the study, and secondly to design the method of data analysis, whether this involves statistics, or the analysis of qualitative data. Where the study may need ethical approval it is worth contacting the appropriate Research Ethics Committee (REC) as soon as possible, as this can seriously delay a study where such committees meet irregularly, or where they have to deal with large numbers of applications. There can also be other stages involved before the ethics committee such as the scientific scrutiny panel that will first assess whether the method proposed is sound. A research proposal, which is the outline of the intended research, will have to be submitted to these various groups, so it is worth getting advice from someone who may have experience in this. Similarly, at this stage advice should be sought from someone who has an understanding of statistics, or the analysis of qualitative data. The method of data analysis will have a profound effect on the type and format of the information included in the data collection tool. A mistake at this point could mean that a large part of the information collected is unusable because it has not been collected in the right way.

Although researchers can spend a great deal of time on planning, and even on piloting the study, it should always be remembered that inevitably things do not always run smoothly, and the unexpected may well happen to you. Research is a skill acquired over time through experience. Don't give up when things go wrong; adjust your plan.

Critiquing research

The research process framework provided in this chapter gives a clear structure to use in evaluating or critiquing projects. As you read through a research report there should be clear evidence that the stages in the research process have been followed, and the issues outlined in this section addressed. If they have not, then you are justified to cast doubt on the way the researcher has conducted the study. Remember, however, that qualitative research has a different structure, and will look different in comparison to quantitative research reports. More details on this will appear in the next chapter.

The important question when critiquing a study is has the researcher followed a sensible plan of action given the nature of the research question?

Following this, the next question should be, does each decision fit with the previous decision made in the process? Once you are familiar with the stages of research you will see the structure clearly evident in the reports you read.

Key Points

♦ Research projects are structured around a number of stages that give the researcher a path to follow. The aim of this framework is to increase objectivity, reliability, validity and the rigour of the research.

♦ The exact sequence of steps will vary depending on the broad research design. Qualitative research is different in structure and process from quantitative.

♦ Knowing these steps enables the reader of a research project to assess whether the correct stages have been followed.

References

Bond S (2000) Preparing a research proposal. In: Cormack D (ed.) The Research Process in Nursing (4th edn). Oxford: Blackwell Science.

Bray J and Rees C (1995) Getting down to research. Practice Nursing 6(8): 18–19.

Brink P and Wood M (1994) Basic Steps in Planning Nursing Research (4th edn). Boston: Jones and Bartlett.

Clegg F (1982) Simple Statistics. Cambridge: Cambridge University Press.

Cluett E and Bluff R (eds) (2000) Principles and Practice of Research in Midwifery. Edinburgh: Baillière Tindall.

Fraser D (2000) Action research to improve the re-registration midwifery curriculum – Part 1: an appropriate methodology. Midwifery 16: 213–223.

Ingram J, Johnson D and Greenwood R (2002) Why are some babies mucousy after birth? British Journal of Midwifery 10(2): 94–98.

Kirkham M (1995) The history of midwifery supervision. In: Association of Radical Midwives (eds). Super-Vision: Recommendations of the Consensus Conference of Midwifery Supervision. Cheshire: Books for Midwives Press.

le May A and Lathlean J (2001) Action research: A design with potential. NT Research 6(4): 502–509.

LoBiondo-Wood G and Haber J (2002) Nursing Research: Methods, Critical Appraisal, and Utilization (5th edn). St. Louis: Mosby.

Moffat H, Lavender T, and Walkinshaw S (2001) Comparing administration of paracetamol for perineal pain. British Journal of Midwifery 9(11): 690–694.

Parahoo K (1997) Nursing Research: Principles, Process and Issues. Houndmills: Macmillan.

Polit D, Beck B and Hungler B (2001). Essentials of Nursing Research: Methods, Appraisal, and Utilization (5th edn). Philadelphia: Lippincott.

Singh D, Newburn M, Smith N and Wiggins M (2002) The information needs of first time mothers. British Journal of Midwifery 10(1): 54–58.

CHAPTER FOUR
Qualitative Research Approaches

There is no one thing that is research; rather, it comes in many shapes, sizes and 'brands'. However, as indicated in Chapter 2, one broad categorization is the distinction between *quantitative* and *qualitative* research approaches. These terms are associated with the types of data produced by each category, but as we shall see later, more fundamental differences lie in the researcher's beliefs concerning the nature of research, and the basic principles they follow in carrying it out.

The amount of research currently available under each of the two headings differs. As Streubert and Carpenter (1999:1) observe, *'the tradition of science is uniquely quantitative'*, and this is equally true of health service research. The development of health care knowledge has conventionally been associated with the 'scientific' image of research. In its crudest characterization, this is often depicted in terms of a frequently male, white-coated figure, working in a laboratory surrounded by test tubes and engrossed in complex numerical calculations. Encouraged by a media thirsty for the 'Gosh' effect of new developments, health service research has been dominated by the dramatic breakthrough in our ability to deal with disease and disability. Interest has centred on life-saving discoveries. This kind of research emphasizes the hard, factual nature of knowledge and the search for objective truth. Even the current emphasis on evidence-based practice is founded on a hierarchy of evidence (Aslam 2000), where the randomized control trial (RCT) has been seen as the 'dependable' way to develop sound practice, because of its emphasis on measurable outcomes.

This leaves qualitative research with many problems, as it has not developed a similar positive and accepted image in the health service. In the past the distinction between 'hard' and 'soft' data, and talk of a quantitative/qualitative 'divide' has exacerbated the view that qualitative research is in some way inferior to quantitative. In reality, it is far better to see these as two distinct approaches to research that answer different types of questions; each having an equal part to play in developing midwifery knowledge and practice.

The aim of this chapter is to restore the balance between the two approaches by concentrating on qualitative research. It will extend the discussion in Chapter 2 by examining some of the main differences between quantitative and qualitative approaches, and describe three major types of qualitative research. The importance of feminist approaches to midwifery will also be emphasized and its relationship to qualitative approaches outlined. We start by outlining the rise of qualitative research within midwifery knowledge and practice.

The rise of qualitative research in midwifery

Historically, there has been a clear difference in medical research, and research carried out in nursing and midwifery. Medicine has embraced the scientific approach of the randomized control trial; midwifery and nursing research, although carried out on a smaller scale, has used a wider range of research approaches. Midwifery has successfully carried out randomized control trials, led either by midwifery researchers alone, or in partnership with others, and has also used surveys to produce descriptive research. Fortunately, there is now a small but growing amount of qualitative research available.

What has qualitative research got to offer midwifery? According to Holloway and Fullbrook (2001) the attraction of qualitative research is its person-centred and holistic approach to generating knowledge. The narrowness of quantitative research means that certain areas of knowledge and understanding are missing, as Holloway and Fullbrook (2001) go on to emphasize:

> When quantative approaches are used there is a danger that researchers miss the rich data which assist in understanding the way people interpret and give meaning to what happens to them, and which enables them to justify their actions.
> (p. 539)

Qualitative research concentrates on an individual's perceptions, experiences, personal insights, beliefs, customs, interpretations of and responses to important aspects of their life, including their health, unusual symptoms, illnesses, and the care they receive from health professionals. It also looks at the same elements from the perspective of health professionals.

The crucial aspect to emphasize is that qualitative research does not concentrate on clinical outcomes, like quantitative research, but rather processes, and our understanding of health and illness issues from the perspective of those involved. It will not give us a clear answer to a clinical problem, but it will help us in our approach to individuals, and groups by providing insights and awareness, rather than remaining in ignorance or under an illusion.

Is this knowledge important to us? How can it not be? Therefore the generation of this knowledge is important within health care if we are to provide a meaningful and appropriate response to health needs. Pregnancy, delivery and childcare are all extremely personal experiences, so any research approach that values human experience will appeal to a profession that emphasizes individuality and an empowering approach to care. Qualitative research, then, is an appropriate choice in exploring some of the important issues facing midwifery.

A further impetus for the growth in qualitative research has been the growing number of midwives attending degree and Masters programmes. This has led to an increased understanding of the available range of research methods. Best-selling research books on these courses have increased the amount of space given to qualitative research over the last 10 years, fuelled by the expanding amount of qualitative research both in America, and to some extent in Britain. Qualitative research articles in journals such as *Journal of Advanced Nursing*, *British Journal of Midwifery*, and *MIDIRS* have also increased and have demonstrated the value of this research approach to the practice of midwifery.

The conclusion to be drawn from this is that all midwives need to be familiar with both quantitative and qualitative approaches to research if they are to demonstrate evidence-based practice. Qualitative approaches balance the narrow focus of quantitative research by examining the bigger picture, and the more human side of service delivery. It does this by exploring the behaviour and perceptions of both women and their families, and of course, midwives themselves. The following section examines some of the major differences between the two major approaches of quantitative and qualitative methods.

The contrast between quantitative and qualitative research

The term qualitative research is a blanket description covering a number of different, but related approaches to research. A simple definition is provided by Langford (2001:137) who describes qualitative research as *'an objective process used to examine subjective human experiences by using non-statistical methods of analysis'*. This neatly sums up the broad characteristics that differentiate qualitative from quantitative approaches. Polit et al (2001) elaborate on this description by outlining some of the key characteristics of qualitative approaches (see Box 4.1).

As these characteristics are important in understanding the differences between quantitative and qualitative research, they require further elaboration.

Qualitative design:

Is flexible and elastic, capable of adjusting to what is being learned during the course of data collection;

Typically involves a merging together of various data collection strategies;

Tends to be holistic, striving for an understanding of the whole;

Requires the researcher to become intensely involved, usually remaining in the field for lengthy periods of time;

Requires the researcher to become the research instrument; and

Requires ongoing analysis of the data to formulate subsequent strategies and to determine when fieldwork is done.

Box 4.1 Characteristics of qualitative approaches to research (reproduced with permission from Polit et al 2001, p. 207)

One way of simplifying this is by demonstrating how the two approaches differ in the following three phases of:

- Planning
- Data collection, including role of the researcher and the nature of the relationship with those involved
- Analysis and interpretation of the results.

Planning

Perhaps the most important characteristic of qualitative research is the holistic approach that attempts to provide a total picture of an individual, their life experiences and beliefs, rather than isolating a single biophysical entity such as temperature, or blood loss. This holistic approach of qualitative research is necessary if it is to achieve its aim of discovering meaning (Burns and Grove 2001). Porter (2000) elaborates on this by suggesting that the uniqueness of qualitative research is that unlike quantitative research it does not focus primarily upon the identification and explanation of facts, but on illuminating people's interpretations of those facts. To achieve this, the research question is broader than that found in quantitative research so that it can capture the bigger picture. The research process followed in qualitative research is also less structured and more flexible, to allow insights during data collection and analysis to develop.

These features have considerable implications for the planning process, which tends to be shorter in qualitative research in an attempt to avoid being 'contaminated' by previous research knowledge. For this reason an in-depth critical review of the literature is often not undertaken at an early stage in the research. However, it is acceptable to undertake a brief overview of the topic through the literature. In the main, however, available literature plays a greater role in data analysis where it is used as a way of confirming the credibility of the researcher's interpretations and descriptions of behaviour. The researcher will include this information along with the data in the findings section. In contrast, quantitative reports do not include the literature in the results section, but do so in the discussion.

A further planning stage distinction is that the qualitative researcher does not develop a structured tool of data collection derived from the literature review, or use a tool that has been validated in previous research. This is because the researcher attempts to keep an open mind on what may be important within the study. The implication of this is that it is not possible to carry out a pilot study, as there is no highly structured research tool to test for reliability. Each interview, or period of observation will be different and not standardized as in quantitative research, which seeks to ensure consistency.

Data collection

In this phase of the research, the researcher may use more than one method of data collection to examine the concept of interest. This is to ensure the use of the best tool for different types of situations, or to confirm the picture emerging from one tool of data collection. Triangulation is therefore a common feature of some forms of qualitative research.

One of the clearest differences between the two research approaches is in the way the researcher forms a relationship with those involved in the study during the process of data collection. As the aim of the research is to gain an understanding and insight into human behaviour, there is an intimacy in the relationship between the researcher and those participating in the research. This mainly develops over a sustained time period not characterized by the quick street interviews or the faceless questionnaire approach. In quantitative research there is traditionally a belief that the researcher should keep their distance from the subjects of the research to avoid undue influence. Although the quantitative researcher is an advocate of 'rapport' with subjects, this does not relate to the same level of intimacy and closeness evident in many examples of qualitative research.

An additional dimension here is where both the researcher and those involved in the research are female. The different styles of interpersonal relationships and communication styles between men and women have long been the subject of popular self-development books (Grey 1993). The more intimate, flexible, and more reciprocal relationship between both parties in qualitative research is far more comfortable and in line with basic personal beliefs for the midwifery researcher. It is also in harmony with the philosophy of feminist research that attempts to minimize any inequalities produced by differences in status between the researcher and those in the research. In fact as we shall see later, there is a close similarity between feminist research and qualitative research.

The nature of this relationship with those in the study means that the researcher has to have a great deal of personal awareness and must make it clear in presenting the findings where the nature of the relationship may have influenced the findings. The impact of the researcher on data gathering has led some commentators to describe the researcher as the tool of data collection or research instrument (Polit et al 2001). By this they mean that so much of the outcome of quantitative research is due to the personal abilities of the researcher to act spontaneously in the way they conduct themselves and how they gather their data.

Data analysis and interpretation

Visually, one of the clearest differences between quantitative and qualitative research is the form of data presentation; the former is presented in the form of numbers and analyzed statistically, and the latter in the form of words and is analyzed in terms of the researcher's interpretation of emerging themes and presented in the form of quotations and descriptions of activities. Streubert and Carpenter (1999) refer to this as a rich literary style.

The relationship between data gathering and analysis is also worthy of note. Unlike quantitative research where the process of data collection and analysis is sequential, in qualitative research the two are carried out in parallel, with data being analyzed during the fieldwork, and this in turn leading to and influencing further data collection. Langford (2001) describes this as a fluid and repetitive process where the researcher is influenced by the unfolding situation. Fieldwork stops when the researcher feels that no new information is emerging and 'data saturation' has been reached.

Analysis in qualitative research is characterized by an *inductive* approach rather than a *deductive* one. This means that the researcher takes the individual elements emerging from the analysis and gradually builds up a picture and broad explanation of what may be going on. In contrast, the quantitative researcher starts with general principles, often in the form of a theory or hypothesis and examines the individual units of data to either confirm or reject that theory or hypothesis.

It is not an exaggeration then, to say that in so many aspects of the research process, the two approaches of quantitative and qualitative are worlds apart. This is illustrated in Table 4.1. Qualitative approaches balance the narrow focus of quantitative research by examining the bigger picture and the more human side of service delivery through the behaviour and perceptions of both women and their families and of midwives themselves. The following section examines some of the more popular qualitative approaches and will illustrate this theme further.

Table 4.1 Summary of differences between quantitative and qualitative approaches

Characteristic	Quantitative	Qualitative
Focus	Narrow and specific	Holistic and general
Research question	Precisely worded	Broadly worded
Nature of the evidence	Objective	Subjective
Belief about reality and research activity	The social world is similar to other 'sciences' and open to measurement by the researcher. Reality is 'out there' and objective	The social world can only be known through an individual's experience and understanding of it. Reality is inside all of us
Researcher's relationship to subjects	Detached to ensure does not influence subjects, although rapport sought	More equal and reciprocal relationship characterized by social warmth
Review of the literature	Critical to the development of the process	Can be used to provide a broad picture, but often used to support findings. It is included as part of written report.
Planning	Carried out in depth	High level of planning avoided so as to reduce preconceived ideas about the nature of the topic

(Continued)

Table 4.1 *(Continued)*

Characteristic	Quantitative	Qualitative
Tool of data collection	Emphasis on accuracy and consistency, to ensure reliability and validity	As the tool is used flexibly and continually developing, it is impossible to pilot to determine consistency and accuracy
Sample size	Emphasis on large numbers to reduce bias and accurately to perform statistical procedures	Small numbers but appropriate experience explored
Sample referred to as	Subjects	'Informants' or 'participants' to avoid dehumanizing
Analytical approach	Deductive	Inductive
Data	Numeric	Words
Data gathering	Extensive to gain maximum coverage	Intensive to gain maximum depth and rich 'thick' data
Product of data analysis	Referred to as 'results'	Referred to as 'findings', although some publications use the term 'results'
Generalizability	Major concern to achieve this to a high level	Not a major concern, low level achieved
Ethical concerns	High, particularly where an intervention is invasive	High, harm is concerned with psychological and social elements and the protection of human dignity
Methodological concerns	Reliability, validity and bias	Trustworthiness, in the form of credibility, dependability, confirmability and transferability
Emphasis on rigour	High	High
Application to evidence-based practice	Highly rated, notably in the form of RCTs	Presently low acceptability, increasing emphasis on user views and experiences may change this
Applicability to midwifery practice	High	High

Qualitative research designs

Although qualitative research can take a vast number of different forms, there are three main categories that dominate; these will be outlined with examples in the following section.

ETHNOGRAPHY

The holistic approach taken by the qualitative researcher is very clearly seen in the work of the ethnographer. Burns and Grove (2001:68) define ethnography as a 'portrait of a people', whilst Donovan (2000:132) describes it as 'a means of obtaining a holistic view of people in their physical and socio-cultural environment and making some sense of their behaviour and inter-action within that setting'. The approach has its roots in anthropology, where the goal of the anthropologist was to describe and interpret activities within a culture or cultural subgroup. These were usually pre-literature and 'exotic' groups where the researcher attempted to learn something about the people and the society as a whole.

Rather than choosing exotic and 'non-literate' tribes, the use of this approach is now applied to everyday cultures, but still with the purposes of understanding the rituals and beliefs that people hold and that influence their behaviour. The underlying assumption of ethnographic research, according to Polit et al (2001:213) is that every human group evolves a cul-ture that guides the members' view of the world and the way they structure their experiences. The authors stress that the aim of the ethnographer is to learn from (rather than to study) members of a cultural group.

The anthropologist's techniques of observation, interviews, participation and immersion in the culture, and the keeping of a fieldwork diary have all been adopted to various extents by the ethnographic researcher in health care. Like the original anthropologists, those undertaking ethnographic research tend to carry out fieldwork for long periods of time in order to observe their chosen group under a range of circumstances. There are dangers in this, as the longer the period of observation the closer and more familiar the relation-ship between the observer and the observed develops. This can lead to what in anthropological studies was called 'going native'. This meant the researcher no longer saw the group's activities through the eyes of an enquiring stranger, but rather as another member of the group with 'taken for granted' or 'tacit' knowledge. To overcome this the researcher attempts to use the tech-nique of 'cultural strangeness'. This means trying to see things as an outsider to the group. This is perhaps one of the difficulties facing the midwifery ethnographer, in that it is very difficult to see things as culturally strange once socialized into the midwifery role.

There are also practical difficulties facing the midwifery ethnographer, particularly the investment of sufficient time to carry out the fieldwork. Polit et al (2001:213) refer to ethnographic research as a typically labour-intensive and time-consuming endeavour. This is because the researcher needs some time to first establish acceptance and a clearly identified role within the group. It is a very intimate relationship where the subjects in the study need to feel comfortable with the researcher and feel they can share deep feelings and shared understandings that they may not want to share with strangers.

Anthropologists are typically concerned with what people do, the objects they make and how they use them, what they say, and how it is said. This helps us understand the way that studies using this approach are structured and the focus of attention. The methods of data collection to achieve these aims typically consist of observation and interviews, both of which tend to be flexible and intense, that is, they are carried out over a long period of time in the field. In some cases other forms of data collection including the use of written accounts, such as records or diaries, are also used to shed light on the situation. In terms of style, the approach of ethnography is very similar to making a 'fly-on-the-wall' documentary. The purpose is not to manipulate a situation, but rather record it and try and make sense of it. Instead of a camera and tape recorder, the ethnographic researcher keeps a 'fieldwork diary' in which they capture the details of their observations, interviews and their personal interpretations and understandings. In presenting their results reference will be made to their fieldwork diary or notes to add detail and accuracy to the observations and interviews.

The following is a useful list of questions that the ethnographer typically tries to answer about the group under study suggested by Langford (2001):

- What procedures does a person follow that makes them a part of a group?
- What practices do group members engage in that result in an end product?
- What kinds of work do members engage in to accomplish the goals of the group?
  (p. 143)

One of the classic ethnographic studies is that of Sheila Hunt (Hunt and Symonds 1995), who set out to explore two maternity units in order to understand the culture, work practices and strategies of midwives. This will be examined later in Chapter 11 on observational methods. Hunt's design is one of triangulation, which uses observation, interviews and a fieldwork diary to make sense of the events taking place in the settings.

PHENOMENOLOGY

Phenomenological research has been influenced by the discipline of philosophy. It attempts to understand the essential nature of people's experiences and interpretations of key features in their life. Most researchers who claim to follow this approach credit the influence of two key philosophers, Husserl, and one of his students, Heidegger, who developed Husserl's ideas in a different direction. Streubert and Carpenter (1999:45) suggest that there were three phases in the development of phenomenological thinking, with a preparatory phase before the German phase dominated by Husserl and Heidegger, and followed by a French phase that included Jean Paul Sartre (1905–1980) and Merleau-Ponty (1905–1980).

The basic purpose of phenomenology is to look at a situation through the eyes of those involved to gain *'the lived experience'* of that phenomenon. LoBiondo-Wood and Haber (2002) describe this approach in the following way:

The phenomenological method is a process of learning and construction of the meaning of human experience through intensive dialogue with persons who

are living the experience. The researcher's goal is to understand the meaning of the experience as it is lived by the participant.
(p. 143)

Ng and Sinclair (2002) provide an example of this in their study that set out to describe the lived experience of a planned home birth. The authors suggest that birth at home is best illustrated by using the metaphor of a woman climbing a mountain, at it symbolizes the essence of the experience. This journey starts from the logical decision to climb the mountain and the preparation for it, the climb up to the summit, which is the experience of the birth, and the events afterwards that form the triumphant descent back down the mountain.

Phenomenological research is typically conducted by means of in-depth interviews. There can be a slight difference of emphasis in studies depending on whether the researcher is following the ideas of Husserl, who concentrated on describing the lived experience. Here, the researcher should put aside their personal understandings, values and preconceptions. This is attempted through the process of *'bracketing'* where the researcher's views are put on one side. Those following more closely the beliefs of Heidegger, do not attempt to bracket; here the focus is on the interpretation of what it is like for those in the study, which is felt to require some prior understanding.

Phenomenology has a great deal to offer midwifery as it provides the perspective of those receiving services and so might open up understandings that may not be available through any other means.

GROUNDED THEORY

This is the most recent approach developed in the 1960s by two American sociologists, Glaser and Strauss as a result of research on hospital staff's behaviour towards dying patients. Although the approach may look similar to either a phenomenological study, or an ethnographic study, the crucial difference is in its purpose. Whereas the aim of the former approaches is to describe by painting a word picture of a situation, the purpose of grounded theory is not only to describe, but also to try and explain, through a proposition of why things might take the form they do. These propositions can be said to form a theory that is 'grounded' in the data collected; thus the term 'grounded theory'.

The method of data collection and analysis is sometimes referred to as a grounded theory approach (see, for instance, Askey and Moss 2001). This usually means that data collection and analysis are carried out in parallel, and stops once 'saturation' occurs, that is no more new analytical categories arise. The analysis also consists of the constant comparison method where new data and emerging categories from the analysis are compared with previous data and categories to ensure consistency and the possible development of links between the categories.

Grounded theory uses such methods as observation alone or with other methods, or interviews. These accord with the previous approaches in being very flexible in design. An important source is also the fieldwork diary in which the researcher keeps a running commentary on the way events unfold and their own reflections and developing understanding of the situation and the topic under consideration.

The main emphasis in the findings section is the development of a model or theory that explains the data collected. This is illustrated in the work of Askey and Moss (2001) who explored the experiences of staff caring for women experiencing a termination of pregnancy for fetal abnormality. They developed a model of what they call 'the evolution of caring', which emerged from their interviews with women. This is shown diagrammatically as a three-stage process comprising 'getting experience', 'learning and developing', and 'experience and maturity'.

Similarly an earlier study by Levi (1999) set out to explore the processes operating and the factors involved when midwives assist women to make informed choices during pregnancy. This resulted in a diagram illustrating the relationship between the main categories arising from the data. This depicts what she calls 'protective steering' where the midwife feels they have to strike a balance between giving enough information to allow women to make a choice, but not give too much information that might frighten them. The paper is illustrated by a cartoon of a midwife walking a tightrope to emphasize the dilemmas faced in providing information.

It is through these conceptual models that midwifery theory can be expanded and practice developed in line with the experiences and perceptions of both midwives and those for whom they care.

Qualitative research within midwifery

The previous sections have indicated how each approach has been applied within midwifery. However, as qualitative research takes so many diverse approaches, not all midwifery research falls neatly into one of these categories. Indeed, as Table 4.2 below illustrates, the researcher may simply state that they have broadly followed a quantitative approach and not specify a particular category. In these instances, the researcher may have followed some of the basic principles of a qualitative approach in valuing the individual's views, experiences or perceptions, or have followed some of the principles of qualitative data analysis to make sense of the findings.

The depth of analysis will also vary from article to article. In some examples the researcher will use a more descriptive approach to presenting the study and summarize the main points made under various headings. Here, the attempt is to paint a picture of the situation from the individual's perspective without attempting to provide analytical comment. These articles can be of practical value, although they might not comply with strict criteria applied to the qualitative approaches described above. In other examples the researcher will provide far more detailed analysis and provide more in-depth 'backstage' information on how the study was carried out and the analysis achieved.

Feminist research

The writer of a qualitative research article will often say they have drawn on a particular approach such as a phenomenology or grounded theory as a

Table 4.2 Examples of midwifery qualitative research

Author and Year	Terms of reference	Stated approach	Sample size	Sampling strategy	Tool(s) of data collection	Method of analysis
West and Topping (2000)	To explore with midwives their perceptions of the use of the policy [of breastfeeding] in practice	Qualitative	10 (Five hospital and community midwives)	Purposive convenience sample	Interviews in focus groups	Kreuger's tape-based analysis
Hanna (2001)	To explore how young women negotiated motherhood and how they constructed their own identities and relationships through teenage parenting	Incorporating ethnographic practices, guided by feminist principles	Five homeless, sole supporting teenage mothers living alone with one or two children	Convenience, contacted through charitable organization	Observation, interviews, field notes, journaling, discussions with key informants	Transcribed interviews and field notes were managed using a data software package (NUD.IST)
Salmon (1999)	To provide an account of women's experiences of perineal trauma in the immediate post-delivery period	Qualitative using a feminist analysis	Six women who had experienced perineal trauma as a result of childbirth	Snowball	Unstructured taped interviews	Feminist analysis guided by an established framework
Ng and Sinclair (2002)	To understand women's lived experience of a planned home birth	Phenomenological	Nine women	Purposive	Interviews	Analysis carried out in keeping with guidelines by Giorgi's method
Shallow (2001a) and (2001b)	To explore midwives' experiences of becoming integrated and how they view working in a team	Modified grounded theory	Six midwives, various parts of an integrated service	Purposive	Interviews	Modified grounded theory was used to analyze the data guided by the work of Strauss and Corbin

part of the methodology section of a research article. This helps the reader anticipate the way the material has been analyzed and the thinking behind that analysis. In midwifery there is a surprisingly small amount of research that states it has drawn on a feminist approach (for example Salmon 1999, Shallow 2001a). As midwives are predominantly female, and the stated aim of midwifery is to be women-centred, it is worth considering why the amount of feminist research in midwifery is so small. The aim of this section is to consider what is meant by feminist research and its relevance to midwifery knowledge.

The starting point is to place feminist research within the context of feminism. As a social movement, feminism takes many forms, but in essence, the ideals of feminism relate to the following three areas:

◆ A valuing of, and emphasis on, the experiences, opinions, ideals and needs of women as a group in society

◆ The oppression of women in society by a dominant male power culture

◆ A desire to improve the position of women in society and the quality of their lives.

Writers such as Kelly et al (1995) state that feminism is based on the belief that gender is a fundamental organizer of social life. In other words, many of the things that happen (or do not happen) to women are because of the way in which males influence all aspects of life to the detriment and disadvantage of women. Men are held to dominate and dismiss the value of women in all spheres of life, even to the extent that they become 'invisible' in the leading decision-making arenas. A major goal of feminism is to raise the profile of women and give them a legitimate voice by redressing the imbalance of power in society. A further goal is the acceptance and legitimization of a female social agenda and an action plan for the issues raised by it. This is seen as a long struggle as it is felt that the negative position of women in society has existed for so long that many women themselves no longer question the disadvantages they face, and have come to see them as 'normal'.

Women's health can be seen as another area in which women are vulnerable and do not always have the power to control the process in which they are involved. Throughout life women's reproductive and general health becomes controlled by medicine. The history of obstetric care is a good example of how a predominantly male obstetric profession has dominated the ideas and discussion on what constitutes a desirable form of service for women during pregnancy and delivery. This has led to some clearly oppressive situations for women in the name of safety and convenience. The quality of the delivery experience and subsequent relationship with their babies has also been influenced by obstetric values and practices. The nature of the interaction between obstetricians has also been seen as problematic. In all of this it is important to recognize that midwifery can find itself supporting a situation that is part of women's powerlessness.

Feminist research developed in response to the dissatisfaction felt by some researchers that the definition of research and the way it was conducted was overly influenced by dominant male researchers. It was felt that the quantitative approach to research neglected answering many of the questions that would benefit women, and feminist research was developed to form a more appropriate approach to addressing these issues.

What is meant by feminist research? Draper (1997:597) suggests the following definition:

> *Feminist research is about making women and their experiences visible. It is concerned not just with researching women, but with the method employed, the philosophical underpinnings to this method and also with practical research 'process' issues.*

This helps to identify the purpose of feminist research and also the processes involved. Again there are a number of different forms that feminist research can take, but a general distinction can be made using the following criteria suggested by Seibold et al (1994), cited in Draper (1997). Seibold suggested that the guiding principles should be:

♦ That women's experiences are the major object of investigation
♦ That the researcher(s) attempts to see the world from the point of view of the women
♦ That the researcher(s) is active in trying to improve the lot of women.

The last point is important as, according to Kelly et al (1995), what makes feminist research is less the method used, but more how it is used and what it is used for. This is supported by Cluett and Bluff (2000) who argue that methods themselves do not appear to have gender, it is the way they are used and the purpose for which they are used.

There are a number of ways in which feminist research parallels the characteristics of qualitative research. These include seeing situations from the individual's (woman's) perspective. However, the philosophical underpinning of the research is based on the principles of feminism. This means that feminist research is carried out with the intention of improving the situation for women. The basic premise of conducting the research and analyzing the results draws very much on an understanding of women's disadvantages in society and their treatment by men.

Unfortunately, this approach has not had a great impact on nursing and midwifery research. Indeed, writers such as Sigsworth (1995) have taken great pains to point out the benefits of feminist research by stressing that it provides a more relevant way of thinking about, and carrying out research, in comparison to the more customary randomized control trial. However, there seems to have been little response to such pleas.

One notable exception is the work of Salmon (1999), who provides an excellent example of feminist research in her study examining women's experiences of perineal trauma. Following six unstructured interviews with women she revealed that a common theme was the negative attitude of the male doctors who had sutured them. The findings point to failure of these doctors to understand women's pain and to acknowledge the severity of the traumatic experience for these women. This leads Salmon to conclude that it is the gendered nature of the relationship between doctor and the women that is largely responsible for the physical and emotional distress felt by the women experiencing perineal trauma. She ends by suggesting that the experiences of these women were shaped by the fact that a man had not understood their needs as a woman at a time of vulnerability.

This work clearly fits the criteria of feminist research in that it values and emphasizes the experiences of this group of women. The situation is outlined through the women's own words concerning the indignities they suffered from the male doctors. Their oppression from the way they were treated and spoken to by these doctors is evident from the interview data. Salmon's rationale in undertaking the research is to raise the issue of the treatment they had received, and to argue that the care of women in this position needs to be improved. It also illustrates how feminist research can make a fundamental difference to the quality of care received by women.

This section emphasizes the way in which research is not just simply a process that is totally objective, but a process that can be used to make a statement concerning a group as a whole, such as women in society. Although the tools employed are similar to those encountered elsewhere, it is the philosophy or values underpinning the way the study was conducted that holds the key. Here it is argued that feminist research has much to offer midwifery research, and at the moment it is grossly underutilized as a legitimate methodology within the profession.

Conducting research

Once the researcher has decided that a qualitative or 'interpretative' approach is appropriate, a decision has to be made on which particular option to select. The research question and purposes of the research will provide some guidance. Questions that consider what it is like to have a certain experience, such as elective caesarean section, or twins, may require more of a phenomenological approach that uncovers the 'lived experience' of individuals. If the question is concerned with behaviours or experiences of an identified group or 'culture' such as midwives, then a more ethnographic approach will be appropriate. If the approach sets out to provide an explanation for a particular activity or belief, such as why do women feel that elective caesarian sections will be an appropriate form of delivery, then a grounded theory approach should be adopted.

Although these different qualitative forms of research were originally very explicitly defined, through use and application within health and other settings, variations and adaptations have arisen. The flexibility of these approaches has sometimes made it difficult to find clearly prescribed procedures for those wanting to carry out this type of research. There is also a lack of learning opportunities to study and practise the techniques of these approaches. For this reason, this type of research is more usually 'informed by' a particular approach rather than following it to the letter.

In the same way that the quantitative researcher must ensure that they fully understand the process of quantitative data collection and analysis, so the qualitative researcher must ensure that their work is carried out rigorously. A number of helpful texts now exist that provide some guidance on the conduct of qualitative research (Holloway and Wheeler 1996, Streubert and Carpenter 1999, Silverman 2000), and how it should be written up (Wolcott 2001). It is advised that potential qualitative researchers study these texts, and participate in courses that specialize in this form of research. The novice qualitative researcher should also read many examples of this type of research in order to get a feel for the way it is conducted and presented.

This is not an easy choice of approach, particularly with phenomenology, because of its history and connection with philosophy. Streubert and Carpenter (1999) recommend that the novice researcher should read some of the original writers of this genre of research such as Husserl, Heidegger, Merleau-Ponty, Spiegelberg, and others, as well as gaining support from a research mentor who will provide advice and guidance on the processes involved. Where possible, try and read articles that describe the researcher's experiences in conducting qualitative research. Hunt and Symond's (1995) work is still a relevant and very readable account of the nature of undertaking qualitative research. Hunt describes in great detail some of the problems, pitfalls and dilemmas she encountered in carrying out her research in a midwifery unit.

As the researcher *is* the method of data collection in qualitative research, it is recommended that they make an attempt to plot their preconceived beliefs about the topic. This plays an important part of rigour in that it allows the researcher to 'bracket' or put aside their beliefs, so that they do not influence the line of questioning or interpretation of what is observed or discussed. In ethnographic research it is recommended that the researcher write a 'fieldwork diary' containing their unfolding thoughts and interpretations. Relevant details from this can be incorporated in the findings of the research to show how ideas and events unfolded for the researcher (Streubert and Carpenter 1999).

Ethical considerations are just as important with this type of research as with quantitative approaches. One added difficulty, however, is that ethics committees may not be familiar with the approach of qualitative research in comparison to quantitative. Some students have, therefore, found it useful to attach brief extracts or explanations of techniques or procedures from research texts as part of a submission.

In carrying out qualitative research one ethical dilemma is the emotional closeness established between researcher and participant. This can lead to details of behaviour or descriptions of events being revealed that might oblige the researcher to break confidence. An example might be a confession regarding conduct towards a child that might be interpreted as putting that child at risk. Under the professional code of conduct a midwifery researcher would have to report that confession or detail. When outlining the nature of the researcher's role, participants should be told that if certain information is revealed to them, the researcher might have an obligation to inform others. Similarly, if the participant seems close to revealing information that might lead to this, they should be reminded of the researcher's duty to break confidences.

It should also be remembered that the nature of qualitative research is very intensive and emotionally challenging. Support from supervisors and personal support can be important in managing the demands that arise.

Finally, if the research question relates to the disadvantage of women during this vulnerable period of their life, and the intention is to reduce this problem, then a feminist approach is relevant.

Critiquing research

The important statement here is that because qualitative research is so different from quantitative research, the same approach to critiquing cannot be used. More details of this will be given in the next chapter on critiquing.

One helpful activity is firstly to confirm that it is qualitative in nature and then to identify which type of approach has been used. Although many research articles contain this information in the title, or at least in the methods section, some authors go no further than stating that their research is qualitative in nature. This means that the method of critiquing can only be broad, and the specific criteria associated with the various approaches cannot be used. However, it is important to satisfy oneself that the common elements that unite qualitative approaches have been satisfied.

As with quantitative research the important question in reading qualitative research is 'can I trust it?' In quantitative research, the key concepts are reliability and validity. It is also important to establish if the research is generalizable. As we shall see in the next chapter, in qualitative research the emphasis is different as the methods of undertaking research follow different principles. The relevant concepts are *credibility*, *auditability* and *fittingness*.

Credibility is concerned with the trustworthiness of the findings. Are they authentic? This is sometimes confirmed either by checking with those who participated in the research that they are an accurate account of the interview or observation; this is called a *'member's check'*. Alternatively, or sometimes in addition, the researcher checks with peers to establish whether others would come to the same conclusions or categories.

Auditability is concerned with the extent to which the researcher illustrates the progress from individual comments or observations to themes. It illustrates how the researcher developed their analysis to show that it is based on an inductive process. Usually in the methods section there will be details on the procedure followed to analyze the findings. This may have the name of someone's approach to analysis such as van Manen, Giorgi, or Colaizzi, all of whom are regularly used as models for data analysis.

Fittingness is concerned with the extent to which the basic principles can be applied to other situations, much as in quantitative research there is an attempt to illustrate the generalizability of the results.

Although many people find that the statistical presentation of results in quantitative research is intimidating, the unfamiliar terminology and thinking behind qualitative research can also be problematic. As qualitative research has a great deal to offer midwifery care, it is important not to be inhibited by the presence of unfamiliar terminology or ideas, rather the reader should identify the underlying messages that can be applied to practice.

Key Points

◆ Qualitative and quantitative research approaches are frequently seen as in conflict with each other, with quantitative research having a long history as 'brand leader' in health care research. In reality, they do different jobs and answer different types of questions.

◆ Qualitative research is interested in illuminating the interpretations and meanings people give to features in their life, including those relating to health. This means that it takes a more holistic and person-centred approach to generating knowledge than quantitative research.

◆ Three major categories of qualitative research are *ethnographic*, *phenomenological* and *grounded theory*. However, many other different approaches exist. All have in common an attempt to see situations through the eyes of those involved. This means that the researcher must attempt to avoid enforcing their own structure and preconceived ideas on the process of data collection and analysis. The issues and themes should emerge from the data collected, which should be directed and controlled as much as possible by those supplying those insights.

◆ Qualitative research is frequently characterized by a close relationship between the researcher and those involved in the study. Indeed, to a very large extent the researcher *is* the tool of data collection in qualitative research.

◆ Issues relating to rigour and ethical considerations are just as important in this type of research as in quantitative research.

◆ Feminist approaches to research contain many of the characteristics of qualitative methods, and seek to improve the situation of women who are disadvantaged by their position as women within health care arenas.

◆ So many elements differ when assessing the two research approaches that it is easy for some people to dismiss qualitative research because of the criteria of evaluating quantitative research they have used.

◆ Midwives need an understanding of both types of research in order to make a balanced approach to evidence-based practice.

References

Askey K and Moss L (2001) Termination for fetal defects: The effect on midwifery staff. British Journal of Midwifery 9(1): 17–24.

Aslam R (2000) Research and evidence in midwifery practice. In: Proctor S and Renfrew M (eds) Linking Research and Practice in Midwifery. Edinburgh: Baillière Tindall.

Bluff R (2000) Grounded theory. In: Cluett E and Bluff R (eds) Principles and Practice of Research in Midwifery. Edinburgh: Baillière Tindall.

Burns N and Grove S (2001) The Practice of Nursing Research: Conduct, Critique, and Utilization (4th edn). Philadelphia: W.B. Saunders.

Cluett E and Bluff R (eds) Principles and Practice of Research in Midwifery. Edinburgh: Baillière Tindall.

Draper J (1997) Potential and problems: the value of feminist approaches to research. British Journal of Midwifery 5(10): 597–600.

Donovan P (2000) Ethnography. In: Cluett E and Bluff R (eds) Principles and Practice of Research in Midwifery. Edinburgh: Baillière Tindall.

Grey J (1993) Men are from Mars, Women are from Venus. London: Thorsons.

Hanna B (2001) Negotiating motherhood: the struggle of teenage mothers. Journal of Advanced Nursing 34(4): 456–464.

Holloway I and Fullbrook P (2001) Revisiting qualitative inquiry: Interviewing in nursing and midwifery research. NT Research 6(1): 539–50.

Holloway I and Wheeler S (1996) Qualitative Research for Nurses. Oxford: Blackwell.

Hunt S and Symonds A (1995) The Social Meaning of Midwifery. Houndmills: Macmillan.

Kelly L, Regan L and Burton S (1995) Defending the indefensible? Quantitative methods and feminist research. In: Holland J, Blair M and Sheldon S (eds) Debates and Issues in Feminist research and Pedagogy. Clevedon: Multilingual Matters Ltd. In association with The Open University.

Langford R (2001) Navigating the Maze of Nursing Research. St. Louis: Mosby.

Levy V (1999) Protective steering: a grounded theory study of the processes by which midwives facilitate informed choices during pregnancy. Journal of Advanced Nursing 29(1): 104–112.

LoBiondo-Wood G and Haber J (2002) Nursing Research: Methods, Critical Appraisal, and Utilization (5th edn). St. Louis: Mosby.

Ng M and Sinclair M (2002) Women's experience of planned home birth: a phenomenological study. RCM Midwives Journal 5(2): 56–59.

Polit D, Beck C and Hungler B (2001) Essentials of Nursing Research: Methods, Appraisal, and Utilization (5th edn). Philadelphia: Lippincott.

Porter S (2000) Qualitative research. In: Cormack D (ed.) The Research Process in Nursing (4th edn). Oxford: Blackwell Science.

Salmon D (1999) A feminist analysis of women's experiences of perineal trauma in the immediate post-delivery period. Midwifery 15(4): 247–256.

Shallow H (2001a) Part 1. Integrating into teams: The midwife's experience. British Journal of Midwifery 9(1): 53–57.

Shallow H (2001b) Connection and disconnection: Experiences of integration. British Journal of Midwifery 9(2): 115–121.

Sigsworth J (1995) Feminist research: its relevance to nursing. Journal of Advanced Nursing 22: 896–899.

Silverman D (2000) Doing Qualitative Research: A Practical Handbook. London: Sage.

Streubert H and Carpenter D (1999) Qualitative Research in Nursing: Advancing the Humanistic Imperative (2nd edn). Philadelphia: Lippincott.

West J and Topping A (2000) Breastfeeding policies: are they used in practice? British Journal of Midwifery 8(1): 36–40.

Wolcott H (2001) Writing Up Qualitative Research (2nd edn). Thousand Oaks: Sage.

CHAPTER FIVE
Critiquing Research Articles

The main purpose of midwifery research is to increase the quality of care through the application of knowledge gained from systematic data collection and analysis. There is a problem, however, and that is the quality of research does vary. We must remember that there is rarely such a thing as the perfect research project. Researchers seldom have ideal conditions in which to carry out their work. One definition of research is that it is making the best of a bad job. But how does the midwife who reads research know what is good, and which should be treated with caution?

Critiquing research is part of the answer. According to LoBiondo-Wood and Haber (2002) a critique is a careful consideration of both the strengths as well as weaknesses of published research. It is on the basis of this that the reader can consider the implications for practice. Although the word critique is often linked with the word criticize, it is meant to be a constructive evaluation, and should be objective, unbiased and impartial. It should take a balanced view of the work in terms of both content and the process of research followed by the author. It is a way of using critical skills to reflect on, not only the whole process in which the research was undertaken, but also the thinking and assumptions on which the research was based.

Critiquing is a skill that requires practice. Firstly, the reader requires knowledge of how to critique. The aim of this chapter is to provide you with that knowledge by providing a structure for critiquing research articles.

As quantitative research is different to qualitative research, the first framework will relate mainly to quantitative research. A second framework for qualitative research will be presented later in the chapter. Some of the details within both structures are based on information in later chapters. This means that you may need to look at later chapters for more detail on some of the points. Critiquing is presented at this point in the book, as it is a skill that should be developed early in learning about research.

As you read this chapter, have a research report that is not too complex by your side. This will help you become familiar with applying the structure of a critique. In the first section you will need an example of a quantitative study, where the results are presented in the form of numbers, and in the second part a qualitative study where dialogue, quotes or descriptions of events are used. There are many examples of quantitative research available, but a good and accessible example of qualitative research would be work on women's experiences of perineal trauma in the immediate post-delivery period (Salmon 1999 or Salmon 2000). More recent work includes Richens (2002) who explored the use of research by midwives, and women's experience of planned home birth (Ng and Sinclair 2002). An excellent longer example of qualitative research is Hunt and Symonds' (1995) ethnographic research on the social meaning of midwifery.

Applying the critiquing framework

When faced with a research article, the reader should consider the following three questions:

1. What does it say?
2. Can I trust it?
3. How does it contribute to practice?

The first question relates to comprehension, and is concerned with such elements as what did they look at? Why did they look at it? How did they go about it? What did they find? What conclusions did they come to? The second question relates to an assessment of the research process in terms of rigour – how well was it thought through, and what steps were taken to reduce problems of bias, reliability and validity? This second question requires knowledge of some of the issues and techniques of research that will be covered throughout this book. The third question relates to an evaluation of the study's contribution to professional practice – does it provide clear evidence for changing or challenging practice? Who might benefit from the study, and in what way?

If we start with the first question of comprehension and what the research says, we might feel that if we read it through we will know what it says. This is not necessarily the case. We know from experience that our reading style may cause us to be selective in what we remember from written material. We will tend to recall unusual or interesting details, or pick out information that reinforces our own views on issues. In other words, our uncritical and unstructured approach to reading may mislead us in our recollections and assessments of written material.

Our very reading style can also make it difficult to accurately assess an article. For instance, have you ever started reading at the top of a page, but by the time you have reached the bottom you have no recollection of what you have just read at the top? If that is a familiar feeling you are in good company. Most of us read passively a great deal of the time. Reading research articles is very different from reading a novel. In fiction the writer is continually drawing pictures in our minds and influencing our feelings, as well as perhaps our senses, with descriptions of sounds, smells and emotions. Research writing is not like that; it requires an approach that is far more active and analytical.

To help us improve our active reading skills and our analytical faculties, we need two things; first of all we need to divide the article into its component parts. This will allow us to see the overall outline of the research, and understand how all the pieces fit together. Secondly, in order to be an active reader it will help us if we have a list of questions to which we can actively search out answers. Box 5.1 provides such a framework and a list of questions. The following sections will now look at these headings in detail.

Focus

When reading a research article the first thing we need to do is identify the broad area it covers, so we can put it in the context of existing knowledge.

1. Focus

In broad terms what is the theme of the article? What are the key words you would file this under? Is the title a clue to the focus? How important is this for the profession/practice?

2. Background

What argument or evidence does the researcher provide that suggests this topic is worthwhile exploring? Is there a review of previous literature on the subject, or reference to government or professional reports that illustrate its importance? Are gaps in the literature or inadequacies with previous methods highlighted? Are local problems or changes that justify the study presented? Is there a trigger that answers the question 'why did they do it then?' Is there a theoretical or conceptual framework that helps us to see how all the elements in the study may be related?

3. Terms of reference

What is the aim of the research? This will usually start with the word 'to', e.g. the aim of this research was to examine/determine/compare/establish/ etc. If relevant, is there a hypothesis? If there is, what are the dependent and independent variables? Are there concept and operational definitions for the key concepts?

4. Study design

What is the broad research approach? Is it quantative or qualitative? Is the design experimental, descriptive or correlation? Is the study design appropriate to the terms of reference?

5. Data collection method

Which tool of data collection has been used? Has a single method been used or triangulation? Has the author addressed the issues of reliability and validity? Has a pilot study been conducted? Have any limitations of the tool been recognized by the author?

6. Ethical considerations

Were the issues of informed consent, confidentiality, addressed? Was any harm or discomfort to individuals balanced against any benefits? Did an ethics committee consider the study?

7. Sample

Who or what makes up the sample? Are there clear inclusion and exclusion criteria? What method of sampling was used? Are those in the sample typical and representative of the larger group, or are there any obvious elements of bias? On how many people/things/events are the results based?

8. Data presentation

In what form are the results presented; tables, bar graphs, pie charts, raw figures, or percentages? Does the author explain and comment on these? Has the author used correlation to establish whether certain variables are associated with each other? Have tests of significance been used to establish to what extent any differences between groups/variables could have happened

Box 5.1 Framework for critiquing quantitative research

by chance? Can you make sense of the way the results have been presented, or could the author have provided more explanation?

9. Main findings

Which are the most important results that relate to the terms of reference? (Think of this as putting the results in priority order; which is the most important result followed by the next most important result, etc. There may only be a small number of these.)

10. Conclusion and recommendations

Using the author's own words, what is the answer to the terms of reference? If relevant, is the hypothesis accepted or rejected? Are the conclusions based on, and supported by the results? What recommendations are made for practice? Are these relevant, specific and feasible?

11. Readability

How readable is it? Is it written in a clear, interesting style, or is it heavy going? Does it assume a lot of technical knowledge about the subject and/or research procedures (i.e. is there much unexplained jargon)?

12. Practice implications

Once you have read it, what is the answer to the question 'so what?' Was it worth doing and publishing? How could it be related to practice? Who might find it relevant and in what way? What questions does it raise for practice and further study?

Box 5.1 (*Continued*)

The focus of an article provides a clue to the general topic. This should be expressed in a few words that include the key concepts covered in the article. These might be found in the title, and most certainly in the terms of reference. Ask yourself what is the basic theme of this article? The answer might be 'empowering women to make informed choice', 'care of the perineum', or 'effectiveness of postnatal visits'. Notice that these are not questions, nor are they long and detailed. We are looking at the broad canvas of which this study forms a part. It should be stressed that sometimes when identifying the focus there is not a clear right or wrong answer, it depends very much on what you see as the basic purpose of the article. Some articles might be put under the focus of 'communication problems', or 'assessing change', while others may be more narrow, such as 'the reduction of pain in labour'.

Background

The background to a study answers the question 'how does the researcher justify choosing this topic area?' Here we should expect to see a clear argument as to why the topic is a problem, the nature and implications of that problem, and how it has been approached in the literature. A study should start with the identification of a problem.

The author may use the subheading *'Review of the literature'* in which previous work will be examined. Some articles will contain only a summary or synopsis of previous work. Where possible, however, an author should provide a critical review of the literature. This should draw attention to both strengths and weaknesses of individual works, and the literature overall. In this section the author may explicitly or implicitly draw together the theoretical or conceptual framework of the study. This will answer the question 'which concepts or variables are seen as linked for the purpose of this study?'

Aim (terms of reference)

The background should prepare the way for the terms of reference that will specify the aim of the study. There are two places where the terms of reference can usually be found. The first is in the summary sometimes found underneath the title, or in the margin in some journals. The second place is just before the subheading 'method'. Although the terms of reference usually begin with the word 'to', sometimes because of the grammatical construction of the sentence we might have to insert it ourselves. If the work is experimental there might also be a hypothesis. Both the terms of reference and hypothesis will be important as our evaluation of some elements of the method, and particularly the conclusion, will be influenced by the author's stated intention of what they wanted to find out, or test.

With the terms of reference and the hypothesis, if present, it should be possible to identify which of the three levels of research questions has been used (see Chapter 2). The variable(s) should also be evident at this stage. Where the question is level three, what are the dependent and independent variables? Has the author provided satisfactory concept and operational definitions for the variables?

Throughout all these sections it is important to keep to the author's own words rather than paraphrase them, as we could change their meaning. In critiquing, it is also important that we are doing two things; we should not only be describing the content under one of the headings in the critique framework, but we should also say how well the author has accomplished that element. In other words it is not simply what they said, but how well they said it.

Methodology

In this section the reader's task is to identify the design of the project, and whether this was a suitable choice to answer the question. The first stage is to identify the broad research approach in terms of – is it:

◆ An experimental design with an experimental and control group?

◆ Correlation where the researcher is searching for patterns between variables, but not as in a cause and effect relationship?

◆ A survey where the purpose is description?

◆ Action research, which involves the introduction of change but with no control group?

◆ Qualitative where the purpose is to gain insights into people's perceptions, beliefs, or behaviour?

The important point here is whether a suitable design has been chosen. Within the broad research approach, which tool of data collection has been used? We should consider some of the strengths and weakness of the method chosen in order to judge whether the author has chosen wisely. Is there recognition of some of the limitations of that method? Has triangulation been applied where the author has used more than one tool of data collection to look at the same variable? We would also consider whether the researcher has attempted to increase the chances of reliability. For instance, have they used a pilot study to check the consistency of the tool of data collection?

The critique includes not only an assessment of the tool of data collection, but the ethical issues related to its use. Here, we are checking to see if informed consent, confidentiality, and an evaluation of the possible negative consequences of taking part in the study have been addressed in the study. Has the researcher gained approval from an ethics committee or is it not appropriate in this case (see Chapter 8)?

We should also look closely at the sample of people, events or objects involved in the study. Are there clear inclusion and exclusion criteria that will help us to consider if they were appropriate for the study (see Chapter 14)? We should also identify the total numbers on whom the results are based. Here, we need to be careful as large numbers could be initially involved, but through a poor response, individuals dropping out, or being eliminated from analysis for one reason or another, the final numbers could be quite small. Our main concern with the sample is whether we feel that it is typical of the group they represent. It is not only sample size, but also geographical variations and characteristics of the sample that we need to think about. Where people are involved, could there be cultural patterns related to the part of the country or social class that might also influence the results?

Main findings

In this section we are concerned with the data the researcher collected, the way it is presented and the extent to which it answers the terms of reference. It is important to make the distinction between the main findings of a study, and what we might think of as interesting findings. We also need to distinguish between the results that relate to the terms of reference, and the purpose they hope to achieve with the results. The main findings answer the research question, the purpose is what will be achieved with the results.

We need to limit our view of the main findings to those results that might have a reasonably large number attached to them, and which relate to the terms of reference. We do have to consider what might be an appropriate or anticipated response to questions or measurements against which we can compare the actual findings. For example, what proportion of women would we expect to have the same midwife present throughout labour? If we would expect in the region of 80%, and the results showed that in only 48% of deliveries did the same midwife attend throughout we would consider this a main finding.

In any study there may only be a small number of perhaps three or four main findings. How easy was it to pick these out?

The results section of studies can look intimidating, especially if we do not have a full understanding of some of the statistical terminology and symbols. However, it does not take long to learn some of these meanings (Clegg 1982), and the results section can become clearer once we have learnt a few of the terms and symbols (see Chapter 13).

Although it is reasonable for authors to make some assumptions about the level of knowledge about statistical techniques readers of certain journals should possess, a reader has the right to feel that certain specialized terms and procedures should be clarified. If the author is interested in reaching the widest audience, then they should explain some of the terms. The author should also explain the tables and graphs, so the reader can follow the reasoning being used to interpret the results. Understanding the results section can take time and perseverance. It is recommended that you refer to some of the more reader-friendly books on statistics, such as the one by Clegg (1982).

In the end

The final part of the critique should look at the conclusion to the study, the recommendations, and then assess the way the study has been presented and the implications for practice. Again, use the author's own words. Following the results of a study the author will present the issues that have arisen from the findings in the discussion. This section may also include the author's own comments on any limitations to the study, such as the size and composition of the sample, or the tool of data collection. These comments should be seen as positive, and part of research rigour, as the researcher is helping the reader to form a balanced view of the results. The discussion section will then take some of the issues or implications raised by the results and put forward the author's interpretation of their relevance for an understanding of the topic. The literature may also be referred to again to underline the extent to which the findings in this particular study are similar to, or different from, those of previous studies. While reading the discussion it is important to consider your own views of the arguments put forward. Do you agree, or are there other possible interpretations?

The final section of a research report should contain a conclusion that provides an answer to the terms of reference. Although there may be a section headed 'conclusion', it may contain only recommendations, or broad statements that do not relate back to the terms of reference. The 'real' conclusion may be found in the discussion. Using some of the words from the terms of reference the conclusion should provide a succinct answer to the terms of reference, or say whether the hypotheses have been accepted or rejected.

Where the terms of reference is made up of more than one part, question or hypothesis, each part should have a clear conclusion. In our assessment, we must consider whether the conclusion was based on, and supported by the results. Given the findings of the study, would we have come to the same conclusion? Is the evidence strong enough to make that conclusion, or are there alternative conclusions that the author has not considered?

The final element may be the recommendations. What does the author suggest could improve the situation? Do these suggestions flow naturally from the discussion? One point to consider is whether the recommendations are realistic and concrete? Are they so vague and general that it is unlikely that improvements could be made? Do they give a clear idea of what it is the reader could go away and do, having read the report?

If we are to produce a critique of an article there are two remaining categories we need to consider. The first is how would we describe its readability? Although research convention dictates the way a study will be reported, this does not mean that it has to be dull and turgid to read. Although we may be more interested in a study that relates to our particular area of work or own interests, any study has the potential to be presented in an interesting way.

We should expect that the research article is written in a clear style, with a minimum of jargon. Complex terminology should be explained or clarified. However, the researcher should expect readers to be familiar with common research terms, and be prepared to look up terms that may be unfamiliar to them, but known to the majority of research readers.

Finally, we come to perhaps the most important section of all, that is the application of the research to clinical practice. Once we have read it, what is the answer to the question 'so what?' We have to think about how the article as a whole may have a message for practice. Is there something that should now happen as a result of these findings? Perhaps we need to consider some of the points in the recommendations to see if there are some things that could relate to our own activities.

Once you applied all the sections in Box 5.1 to an article, you should feel that you have a clear understanding of how the author carried out the study. You should also feel that you have not accepted the author's work uncritically. Critiquing a research article is a meeting of minds; the researcher's and yours. The result should be a greater understanding and consideration of the topic under study.

Critiquing a research article should not automatically result in change. It may take other similar studies to produce a sufficient weight of evidence to suggest changes in practice. A single study, however, could make us question what we do, and its effectiveness. We might start to think whether some of our knowledge has passed its 'sell-by-date' and whether we need to look at our practices more critically.

If we have conducted the critique fairly, we should be able to evaluate research from a more informed and objective standpoint, and not reject it simply because it does not agree with our own views on the subject. Midwifery needs its practitioners to exercise this skill for the benefit of all

1. Focus

What is the key issue, concept or problem that this work examines? What are the key words you would file this article under? Are there clues to the focus in title? How important is this for practice and the profession?

2. Background

What argument or evidence does the researcher provide for exploring this issue, concept or problem? Is there a review of previous literature on the subject or reference to government or professional reports that illustrate its importance? Are gaps in the literature or inadequacies with previous methods highlighted? Does the literature review examine the concepts or issues that form the focus? Is there an attempt to justify the study within the context of a qualitative research design? If this is grounded theory there may not be a comprehensive review of the literature at this point, although some reference to previous work may be presented as an illustration of its importance. There should be some argument or background information to justify looking at this particular subject.

3. Terms of reference

What is the stated aim of the research? This will usually start with the word 'to'. There will not be a hypothesis or the identification of dependent and independent variables, as qualitative research answers a level 1 question. There may be an attempt to provide a concept definition for the concept that forms the focus of the study. On the whole you will find the terms of reference are very broad and general and not as specific as quantitative research.

4. Study design   Page 27

There may be an acknowledgement that the study is qualitative and then a statement made on the specific approach that has been used. The main alternatives are i) phenomenological, which explores what it is like to have a certain experience such as a delivery, a pregnancy or threatened miscarriage, and how people interpret that experience; ii) ethnographic, where the researcher enters and participates in the world of the subject by listening, observing and asking questions in order to understand their view of the world, or iii) grounded theory, which will identify concepts which arise from the analysis of the data collected, and may also suggest a theory or hypothesis that explains or predicts relationships between some of the concepts that have emerged in the study. It is important that the philosophy behind the method suits the intentions of the research.

5. Tool of data collection   Page 28

Here we are interested not only in the technique used to collect the information, but the amount of detail we have on the circumstances under which the data were collected. This contributes to the credibility of the study. This should include details of the environment in which the data were collected, over what period of time data collection took place, and any other details that allow us to visualize the conduct of data collection. Did the researcher spend sufficient time, either in observing the life and behaviour of the subjects, or in interviewing subjects, to produce sufficient depth to the data? Because of the flexible

Box 5.2 Framework for critiquing qualitative research. (It is suggested that you photocopy this box, and use alongside relevant articles)

way that data are gathered, and the way the method will change during data collection, a pilot study will not usually be employed. The researcher should, however, include detail of how they have attempted to achieve procedural rigour in the way the study was conducted. Did they check with those in the study that the information collected was accurate (member's check)?

6. Ethical considerations   Page 29

As with qualitative studies, it is important that the researcher has protected the participant from harm, and has gained informed consent from those taking part in the study. It should not be possible to identify individuals or places where the study took place where this might affect anonymity. The researcher should illustrate ethical rigour, including where appropriate approaching a Research Ethics Committee (REC), or in American studies an Institutional Review Board (IRB), to approve the research.

7. Sample

Who makes up the sample and what are their basic characteristics? The sample size may be quite small, even down to 3 or 4, but more usually about 10 to 12. This may be dictated by theoretical saturation, that is, data collection stops once there is repetition in the type of information or categories emerging. In qualitative research it is important to assess whether the participants possess the relevant knowledge or carry out the activity in which the researcher is interested. Has the researcher demonstrated that the participants are able to provide relevant information and are not open to any kind of bias? The reader must consider to what extent the findings, theory or conceptual categories may apply to other settings. This contributes to its fittingness to be applied elsewhere.

8. Data presentation   Stage 5/6. page 30

The data will be presented in the form of description, dialogue or comments from participants. Is this 'thick' and 'rich' description? Is there sufficient detail for us to almost feel that we are there? Do the quotes from participants clearly illustrate the concepts they are being used to illustrate? Is there over-dependence on comments from a small number of the participants in the sample? Has the researcher detailed how they ensured that the data were accurately recorded and representative of the data gathered? Is there anything about the circumstances in which the data were collected that could have threatened the accuracy of the data? Is it possible to discover the 'decision trail' used by the researcher to determine how the raw data was processed into the categories presented in the results section? This contributes to its auditability. Given the same data it should be possible, following the decision trail, to arrive at similar categories and conclusions. Does the researcher present the findings in the participant's own words rather than reinterpreting what was said or done?

9. Main findings

What are the key concepts or categories developed from the data? Do the concepts and categories presented cover all the data gathered? Were the findings checked either by the participants (members check) or examined by other experts in the field? Are the main findings credible, that is, have attempts been

Box 5.2   *(Continued)*

made to support the accuracy of the results through rigour in the way in which the study was conducted? Does the researcher discuss the findings and relate these to the literature, or do they appear to believe that the quotes will speak for themselves?

10. Conclusion

Is there a clear answer to the terms of reference? Does the researcher propose a relationship between the concepts and categories developed in the analysis to form a clear conceptual or theoretical framework? Does the conceptual or theoretical framework reflect the data? Has the conclusion been arrived at inductively (built up from the findings)?

11. Readability

Does the researcher present the description of the social circumstances described in the research in sufficient detail that one can almost imagine being there, and hear the participants talking and carrying out the activities described? Is it possible to recognize the concepts described as related to practical experience? Is the way the report is written clear and understandable? Is there a clear 'story line' emerging from the research?

12. Relevance to practice

Are the findings relevant to practice or professional knowledge? Is it an important area related to current concerns and issues within the profession? Does the research satisfy the criteria of transferability, that is, can the findings in the form of the theory, concepts or categories developed through the study be applied to other situations, or are they only applicable to the place and the people where the study took place? Do you feel the research has sensitized you to issues or provided further insight? Has it confirmed views you might have already held?

Box 5.2 (Continued)

concerned. However, as a skill it does need practice. As you work through this book, you will gain more and more knowledge that can be applied when critiquing. It is immensely helpful if you can discuss your critique with others who have similar or more advanced skills in this. You should find that once you have used the framework for some time, you will begin to use it in your mind almost automatically, and you will not need to draw on the printed structure. You will then have reached the point where you have become an analytical consumer of research.

Critiquing qualitative research

The aim of qualitative research like that of quantitative research is to increase our knowledge, and so improve practice. As a number of areas important to midwifery do not lend themselves to numeric results and statistical accuracy, other methodological approaches are applicable. Qualitative research is one such alternative (see Chapter 4).

There are a number of different categories of qualitative research, but Holloway and Wheeler (1996) suggest that they have the following basic principles in common:

◆ They take the point of view of the subjects of the research. This is called 'the insiders' or 'emic' perspective

◆ Researchers immerse themselves in the setting and involve themselves with the subjects and the culture to which they belong

◆ Data are not collected according to a predetermined theoretical framework, but the reverse; the data are used to develop a theory

◆ The researcher provides 'thick' description of the way the study was undertaken, this describes what took place in the study in sufficient depth for the reader to almost experience for themselves what it was like in that setting

◆ The relationship between the researcher and those in the study is close and is one of equality and respect

◆ Analysis takes place at the same time as data collection.

These features emphasize the differences in the way the research is conducted and presented, and illustrate why the use of the critiquing framework in the previous section to qualitative research articles is not just difficult, but in many ways inappropriate. Any attempt to use the quantitative approach to critiquing would inevitably lead to unfair criticism, as the way qualitative research is conducted appears to break many of the principles of quantitative research. These includes such things as establishing 'scientific' (i.e. measurable) objectivity and the maintenance of social distance between the researcher and those involved in the study to avoid bias and 'contaminating' the results. From a midwifery point of view an approach that concentrates on understanding and insight seems eminently suitable and compatible with a woman-centred focus of care.

Although qualitative research is similar to quantitative research in its desire to be accurate and rigorous, we need to adapt the critiquing framework to take account of the different principles and philosophy of the approach. In this section some of the essential features of qualitative research are outlined and are related to a framework for critiquing qualitative reports (see Box 5.2).

Focus, background and aim

Qualitative research identifies a particular problem that needs exploring and this centres on a key concept, issue or theme. As with quantitative research, the researcher should provide a clear rationale as to why the study has been undertaken. This will consist of the identification of important professional issues, local details, or key concepts relevant to the profession or clinical practice. These key concepts should be clearly defined in the background to the study. In the case of some forms of qualitative research, such as grounded theory, the researcher avoids reading too much literature prior to data collection. This is in case it influences the way the data are collected and prejudges what are deemed to be important issues. In preference, the researcher will allow participants to define the important issues. Other forms of qualitative research may present a critical review of the literature, in the same way as quantitative studies. The researcher will state the terms of reference, but this may be deliberately broad to provide flexibility and avoid preconceived ideas. It may well simply say the intention is to examine the experience or perception of some concept or other.

Methodology

In outlining the methodology, the researcher should be as rigorous as the quantitative researcher, and illustrate the steps taken to make the process of data collection as accurate as possible. As an attempt is made to avoid separating subjects from the social contexts in which they function, there should be rich or 'thick' descriptions of the setting. Holloway and Wheeler (1996) suggest that 'thick' description involves detailed portrayals of the participants' experiences, going beyond a report of surface phenomena. It involves details of the location and the people within it, thus providing a very visual picture of what is going on. This should be so detailed that we almost feel ourselves to be there. A lack of 'thick data' results in 'thin data' where there is only a surface impression that lacks detail and interpretation.

As the researcher attempts to be as flexible as possible in collecting the data and will attempt to analyze the data at the same time as collecting the data, there will rarely be a pilot study. This brings into question the issue of the reliability of the data collection tool. Whereas the quantitative researcher is influenced by reliability and validity, according to LoBiondo-Wood and Haber (2002) the concerns of the qualitative researcher are *credibility, auditability* and *fittingness*. Credibility relates to the extent to which the researcher tries to ensure the accuracy of the results, auditability relates to the extent to which the researcher provides details on how categories were developed from the data collected, and fittingness relates to the extent to which the results are applicable outside the specific context in which the study was undertaken.

The sample size of qualitative research tends to be much smaller than quantitative research as data collection is a more lengthy process. The aim is not to produce a sample that is statistically similar to the larger population; the intention is to include those in a position to talk in an informed way about the concept of concern to the study. In qualitative research the researcher is often dependent on 'informants' who volunteer information, or agree to provide an insider's view of things. We should expect, however, that there is an attempt to acknowledge and limit bias as much as possible so that the range of experiences or opinions is covered by the sample. Once the researcher feels that subjects are repeating what has already been revealed, they may end data collection on the grounds that 'saturation' has been reached, and further participants would not add anything new to the study.

The issue of ethics should also be addressed, as they are just as important in this type of research as in any other. Here the researcher attempts to ensure that the individual is not put at any disadvantage as a result of being part of the study and should gain informed consent from participants. Where appropriate the Research Ethics Committee (REC) will also be approached to give approval for the study. American studies will refer to an Institutional Review Board (IRB), which serves the same purpose.

Analysis

It is true to say that the crucial part of qualitative research is the analysis. At this point the researcher inductively analyzes the findings for what they might reveal about the subject of the study. If the researcher is to avoid the accusation of subjectivity, they should make it clear how decisions have been made throughout the research so that the reader can understand the thinking employed, not only in conducting the research, but also in the analysis of the findings. This should take the form of a 'decision trail' for the reader to follow.

The results section of qualitative research is frequently referred to as the 'findings', and differs from that of quantitative research, as it will take the form of quotes, either from a participant, or dialogue involving both a participant and the researcher. It may also include descriptions of places, or events. In some instances, these will be extracts from the researcher's *'fieldwork diary'* or notebook.

Morse and Field (1996) warn that it is not enough to simply present dialogue or quotes in the findings section, as the researcher must be more than the editor of an audiotaped story. They suggest that the comments surrounding quotations in the text should be thoughtfully rediscussed and brought to a general level of discussion and not left to 'speak for itself'. Along with the presentation of this form of data, the findings section may also include reference to the literature, which is used as part of establishing credibility for the results of the study, as well as contributing to the analysis of the data.

Conclusion

The conclusion of the study may not only include the answer to the terms of reference, but may also put forward a possible explanation regarding the focus of the study and suggest some relationship to other variables. This may also result in the statement of a theory, or a conceptual framework that may be explored through subsequent research.

Application to practice

The reader of qualitative research will want to draw out the relevance of the research for practice, and the profession as a whole. As one of the aims of qualitative research is to sensitize the reader to the position of those in the study, the application to practice will include the extent to which new insights and awareness have been achieved through reading the study. Although it is often assumed that the findings of qualitative research are not generalizable, Morse and Field (1996) make the point that it is the theory and insights established by the study that are applicable to other situations. The rigour relating to the way in which the research has been conducted will also be brought into question at this point, as the accuracy of the findings must be considered, and the extent to which any theoretical or conceptual frameworks really do fit the situation described.

This outline of the framework for qualitative research indicates that this form of research is no less rigorous than other forms. The way in which the reader approaches the published work is no less systematic than any other study. Although the research can appear very descriptive it can be as beneficial to practice as experimental research. This is because it can provide insights into practice and experiences that may not be possible for the individual midwife to access and so provide a more informed and sensitive approach to care.

Conducting research

There are two reasons why this chapter is relevant to those undertaking research. Firstly, the skill of critiquing is an essential part of reviewing the literature, and therefore the researcher should approach the literature in a critical and analytical way. Henceforth, the methods outlined here are important for the researcher to apply when considering the work of others.

Secondly, the researcher should remember that at the conclusion of their study a report will be written, and perhaps an article published. These will be subjected to the type of scrutiny suggested here. If the researcher is aware of the criteria and framework that readers will use to evaluate their work, then they can ensure that these areas are addressed when communicating the study.

In this section on qualitative research, it has been emphasized how important it is for the researcher to paint a very clear and vivid picture of their experience in conducting the study. This process is facilitated through the use of a fieldwork diary, or field-notes (Polit et al 2001). These should contain all the essential descriptive elements relating to the fieldwork. In the same way they should also contain the major analytical processes that unfolded throughout data analysis. It is from these that the researcher can clearly describe their decision trail and illuminates how the different conceptual categories arose from the mass of findings.

Critiquing research

This chapter has emphasized the need to question and critically analyze published research. If practice is to be evidence-based it is necessary for all practitioners to develop analytical skills. This should not be a purely negative activity, but should take a balanced view identifying both the strengths and weaknesses of the work examined. Remember, research is a difficult activity and it is important to identify the limitations of a study whilst recognizing the constraints under which research is conducted.

Critiquing is a skill, and as such requires practice. It is useful if discussion on research articles takes place between practitioners. These can be on an informal basis, or on a more formal level, as in the case of journal clubs and research interest groups. In either context it is important to be systematic in the way the critique is conducted. It is also important that the appropriate critiquing format has been used on the research. There is no use applying the quantitative critiquing framework on a qualitative article. This chapter has attempted to provide a suitable framework in order for you to critique articles, and research reports. You might find it useful to photocopy the two tables so that you have a more readily accessible checklist to follow when critiquing.

Key Points

♦ A researcher rarely has the ideal conditions under which to conduct research, and so weaknesses can be found in most published research. Just because a piece of research has been published does not mean it is above constructive criticism.

♦ In order to critique an article it is important to use a systematic approach. This chapter has provided two critique frameworks: one that can be applied to quantitative research articles, and one that can be applied to qualitative research. As quantitative research is based on completely different principles from those of qualitative, it is important that the criteria for judging one are not applied to the other.

♦ A critique should have a balance between description – what the researcher(s) did, and analysis – how well it was done. It is not a negative criticism of a piece of research, but should recognize strengths, as well as limitations. Undertaking a critique provides a sound basis for establishing research-based practice, as it ensures that published research is carefully evaluated and not accepted on face value.

References

Clegg F (1982) Simple Statistics. Cambridge: Cambridge University Press.

Holloway I and Wheeler S (1996) Qualitative Research for Nurses. Oxford: Blackwell Science.

Hunt S and Symonds A (1995) The Social Meaning of Midwifery. Houndmills: Macmillan.

LoBiondo-Wood G and Haber J (2002). Nursing Research: Methods, Critical Appraisal, and Utilization (5th edn). St. Louis: Mosby.

Morse J and Field P (1996) Nursing Research: The Application of Qualitative Approaches (2nd edn). London: Chapman and Hall.

Ng M and Sinclair M (2002) Women's experience of planned home birth: a phenomenological study. RCM Midwives Journal 5(2): 56–59.

Polit D, Beck B and Hungler B (2001). Essentials of Nursing Research: Methods, Appraisal, and Utilization (5th edn). Philadelphia: Lippincott.

Richens Y (2002) Are midwives using research evidence in practice? British Journal of Midwifery 10(1): 11–16.

Salmon D (1999) A feminist analysis of women's experiences of perineal trauma in the immediate post-delivery period. Midwifery 15(4): 247–256.

Salmon D (2000) A feminist analysis of women's experiences of perineal trauma in the immediate post-delivery period. MIDIRS Midwifery Digest 10(2): 219–225.

CHAPTER SIX
Reviewing the Literature

A review of the literature can be defined as the critical examination of a defined selection of published literature on a particular topic or issue. Carnwell and Daly (2001) maintain that conducting and constructing a review can be one of the most challenging aspects of the research process, and one where many researchers and students have experienced difficulty. It is not simply a task carried out by researchers, but has now become an important part of clinical practice in relation to clinical effectiveness and evidenced-based practice, and is a familiar activity in many course assignments. The aim of this chapter is to help overcome some of the difficulties by providing practical advice on producing a critical review of the literature that can be used in many types of situations.

There are perhaps four main reasons for carrying out a review of the literature; two relate to clinical uses, and two to academic uses (Figure 6.1). Firstly, it is part of the research process where its purpose is to inform the researcher on the present state of knowledge on the topic to be covered by the study. Any research project should be placed within the context of previous research, so the review of the literature is the method by which this is achieved. It also provides the researcher with valuable information on the methods used in previous studies that might influence the present approach. From this the researcher can learn which approaches are conducive to answering the research question, and which may present problems to overcome.

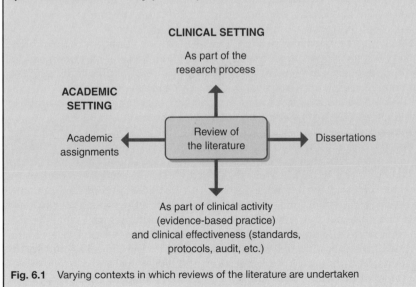

Fig. 6.1   Varying contexts in which reviews of the literature are undertaken

Secondly, a review of the literature is an important element in clinical effectiveness where clinicians search for evidence of best practice on which to base clinical decisions. The review can be conducted and used by an individual practitioner to inform evidence-based practice. It can also play a crucial role in clinical effectiveness where a group of staff in a clinical area seeks to establish clinical standards that can be audited and constructs clinical protocols that will inform the practice of all those in that clinical area. This kind of review can also be used as part of deciding wider policy within a clinical area.

If a review of the literature is to inform practice by suggesting 'best practice', it has to achieve certain standards. So, for example, it should be a critical review of up-to-date research and should be as complete as possible. In addition, those undertaking the review should weed out poorly conducted research that might adversely influence the conclusions of the review and strive to ensure that only the best information is collected, evaluated and included in the review. This in essence is the role of the *systematic review of the literature*. Parahoo (1997) emphasizes the importance of this type of review when he points out that systematic reviews are central to the drive for evidence-based health care. The key is to avoid missing any important studies by only drawing on those that are readily available, as these may be far from representative. Hek et al (2000) make an important point in relation to systematic reviews when they say:

> *Systematic reviews endeavour only to include studies which have low susceptibility to bias, and randomized controlled trial (RCTs) are the preferred design to include because they provide reliable estimates of effect.* (p. 41)

Here we can see the key to systematic reviews is to concentrate on randomized control trials because of the high level of reliability and validity that comes with them. The problem within midwifery, as with nursing, is that so little research produced within midwifery comes under this heading because of the broad nature of midwifery research and the difficulties encountered by those not in medicine to gain funding for this type of endeavour.

Finally, in the academic setting a review of the literature is a frequent activity within many courses of study, either as an integral part of an assignment, or as the main focus of an assignment or dissertation. Indeed, in the past one of the main reasons for undertaking a review of the literature was to fulfil the obligations of a course assignment; anyone carrying out a review was immediately identifiable as a student on a course!

The approach to the review will be slightly different within each of these four activities, and the skills required will also vary. The main differences will be in the extent of the search of the literature included and the depth of critical analysis. The focus will also vary, in that where the review is a part of the research process, the emphasis will be on both the findings of previous research, and the methods employed. This is so that the researcher can learn from the processes that others have used to carry out research in that particular topic area, and so inform their own approach. In the clinical area, the review of the literature will focus more directly on the clinical application of the material, although those undertaking the review will still critically examine the methods used to generate the knowledge to ensure that it has been the result of a rigorous process.

In the academic setting, the depth of analysis will vary with the academic level of the course. Most levels now encourage critical analysis and not just the summarizing of material. At dissertation level, the depth of analysis will be paramount and the research knowledge of the student should be clearly illustrated. The dissertation will also concentrate on a far greater conceptual or abstract level of analysis, often relating the literature to a theoretical or conceptual framework.

All these forms of the review will have certain core features illustrated in this chapter. Certainly, the process of reviewing the literature has become more sophisticated with a greater emphasis placed on explicit details of the search mechanisms employed and the demonstration of rigour in the way the process has been conducted.

In this chapter we shall concentrate on the review as part of the research process, but keep in mind that the skills outlined can be transferred to, and will form an essential part of their use in other settings.

The purpose of a review of the literature is not merely to summarize the published work of others. This is clearly illustrated in the range of purposes of the review suggested by LoBiondo-Wood and Haber (2002), where a review of the literature:

1. Determines what is known and unknown about a subject, concept or problem.
2. Determines gaps, consistencies and inconsistencies in the literature about a subject, concept or problem.
3. Discovers unanswered questions about a subject, concept or problem.
4. Discovers conceptual traditions used to examine problems.
5. Uncovers a new practice intervention(s), or gains support for current intervention(s), protocols, and policies.
6. Promotes revising and development of new practice protocols, policies, and projects/activities related to nursing practice.
7. Generates useful research questions, projects or activities for the discipline.
8. Determines an appropriate research design, methodology and analysis for answering the research question(s) or hypothesis(es) based on an assessment of the strengths and weaknesses of earlier work.
9. Determines the need for replication of a study or refinement of a study.
10. Synthesizes the strengths, weaknesses and findings of available studies on a topic/problem.
    (p. 79)

This list is useful in providing a checklist of some of the elements we should include in our own reviews and what we should look for in those of others.

The process of reviewing the literature

There is a clear process that should be followed in order to produce a rigorous review of the literature. This consists of the following three

- *What* (definitions of key terms or concepts)
- *Why* (what are the causes/influences of the key term/concept)
- *Who* (is particularly affected/at risk/involved)
- *When* (are there particular times when this might happen or action ought to be taken)
- *How* (does it happen/take place/can we do something about it)
- *Problems*
- *Solutions/recommendations*
- *Advantages*
- *Disadvantages*
- *Implications for practice.*

Box 6.1   Key words that may help to identify suitable theme headings for structuring a review

broad stages, each with its own demands and skills required to accomplish them:

- Searching for and locating appropriate literature
- Critically examining the results and extracting relevant detail
- Synthesizing and writing the review.

There are clear similarities between conducting a review of the literature and a research project; both start with a clear question, and maximum effort must go into the planning stage. It is no use saying, 'I want to find out about women who have twins'. To be successful, you have to be clear on why you are carrying out the review, and think what questions you want the review to answer. A more suitable question would be 'What are the main physical, psychological and social problems faced by women who have twins?'

The aim of the review should be specific, and may consist of a number of subheadings under which you will group the literature. The key words that may prompt you to clarify the headings under which the review will be structured are listed in Box 6.1.

Not all of these would be used for every subject. If we take an example of reviewing the literature on twins discussed above, we can see how they can be applied in practice. The process of planning the review may follow similar lines to that outlined in Box 6.2.

If at this stage it is clear that the review is going to be large the scope can be reduced to look at an aspect of it, such as looking at the consequence of twins in the first six months following delivery. In this way the planning stage helps to clarify the question the review will answer. It is also important to realize that some of the above questions will vary in emphasis. This will have implications for the amount of space devoted to exploring it. The answers to some questions will be discussed in a sentence or two; others will be several pages long.

As the review progresses, it may be decided to put some of the material such as the 'what is meant by' in the introduction to the review, and theme

Aim of the review:

To consider the physical, psychological and social implications of the birth of twins on the mother and family, and to identify the implications of these factors for the midwife.

Possible theme headings:

◆ *What* are twins – how is this clinically defined, what variations are there?
◆ *Why* do twins occur – what are the factors associated with twin pregnancies?
◆ *Who* is most likely to have twins?
◆ *When* should some of the implications he considered?
◆ *How* do twins influence physical, psychological, social factors related to the mother and family?
◆ *Problems* – what problems are associated with twins in pregnancy, delivery, and early months?
◆ *Solutions* – how can some of the identified problems he reduced?
◆ *What* are the *implications* for the midwife?

Box 6.2   Planning a review of the literature

the main sections on the issues of problems and solutions. Some of the shorter sections may also be 'collapsed' to form a more substantial section. As a suggestion, the main section of the review should be written under about three to five theme headings, but this is only a very general guideline.

Finding the literature

We are now in a position to think about finding the literature. In the main, reviews of the literature are concerned with information available in journal articles. This is because journals are usually more up to date than books. This may not always be the case, as books now seem to be produced very quickly, especially those linked to disasters, public events and scandals. On the other hand, some journals can take over a year to publish an article. Look at the 'acceptance date' on articles in some journals and you may be surprised at the length of time it has taken to publish them. There may, therefore, be some information included from books in reviews, but they do tend to form a small part of the final work.

In finding what has been produced, the first place that springs to mind to start the search is a library. Nowadays, most health libraries of any size, particularly if they have an educational function, have a computerized index system on a CD Rom containing databases such as CINAHL (Cumulative Index for Nursing and Allied Health Literature). These hold details of published articles on a wide variety of topics. In addition many libraries may also provide access to the Internet that also has links to other databases. These facilities illustrate the way that libraries have changed over the last ten years, and they will continue do so. Hart (1998) draws attention to these changes by saying that many academic libraries have become gateways to information rather than storehouses of knowledge. However, as facilities available on home computers continue to expand, soon we will be able to carry out a great deal of this activity in our own home instead of accessing library buildings that may be geographically some way from us, and open at inconvenient times. In the ideal world, databased material should be readily available in the clinical area where midwives will be able to access complete information to download and use as part of evidence-based practice.

Wherever they are located, databases will need a *key word*, or key words to be typed in, before they are able to provide a list of articles with those words in the title or summary of the article. The problem is frequently finding the right word under which appropriate articles are stored. So for instance 'parentcraft' may not work but 'antenatal education' might.

In writing a review of the literature it is now usual to name the databases used, the key words used to find the literature, any inclusion/exclusion criteria for articles (e.g. only UK articles, or only midwifery sources), and the time frame used to search (how far back your search extends, e.g. five or ten years). Some advanced articles also include the number of articles found ('hits') in various databases, and the numbers rejected for whatever reason. It is important then, to record these details so that if required, you can clearly demonstrate how you arrived at the articles included in your study. The idea is that you should present sufficient information for someone to follow reasonably closely in your footsteps.

Once the database has identified some likely titles, it is a case of locating them. This is where the problems frequently begin. The list of articles may include many references to articles in journals not stocked by your library. Although it is sometimes possible to order them through inter-library loan, this can be costly. Some libraries can be reluctant to supply above a certain number of inter-library loans, as they are costly to their budget, so it is worth ensuring that articles are likely to be essential to your review before ordering. Where the library does stock the journal there can still be a number of problems, these include:

- The library does not have the journal for that time period
- All the copies of a particular journal are there apart from the one you want
- The library has the journal somewhere, but a complete search of the shelves and desks fails to locate it
- The copy you want is there, but when you open it the pages you want are missing.

For these reasons it is important to avoid depending solely on this source of information in the library. Polit et al (2001) warn that locating relevant literature is a skill that requires adaptability. They suggest that locating relevant information on a particular topic is a bit like being a detective, as it inevitably requires some digging for, and a lot of sifting and sorting of clues as to where information is hidden.

One useful technique in searching for clues is *'backward chaining'*. This involves finding one article relevant to your topic and checking their list of references. This will help to locate other similar articles. The reference lists of these articles are then checked for further suitable articles, and so on. Once this has been completed several times you should find the same names keep cropping up. These are the references you must try and locate, as they are the ones that play a major part in our understanding of the topic.

There is one major problem with backward chaining and that is the article you use as a starting point. If this is some years old, you will be backward chaining into a period where the information may have passed its 'sell-by' date. One way to avoid this is by incorporating backward chaining into another good method. This is *browsing* the journal shelves and, using likely journals, going through recent copies for a 'starter' article from which you can backward chain.

At the end of this stage of searching the literature, the reviewer may be faced with one of two problems to overcome. The first is a shortage of likely references, that is, there are very few 'hits'. It is worth checking that the right search terms have been used. The problem may be no more than a typing or spelling error. If the word appears correct, then it could be that the database keeps the information under a different key word. Try an alternative word. Asking library staff for suggestions may be useful, or if you have any articles at all under the subject, check if they list key words that the article has been listed under and try those. If this still does not produce many references, you may need to broaden the topic out to include a wider subject of which your key word may form a part.

The second problem you may be faced with is the opposite of the above, where you have far too much information. Here, you may have to limit the search in some way. One alternative is to reduce the time frame covered by the review to a smaller number of years. You could also try to reduce the topic by taking one particular aspect of it rather than the whole topic. So if you are looking for information giving, you may limit it to the antenatal period rather than information giving in general.

Before we leave this section, it is important to recognize that not everyone feels comfortable and at ease working in a library. The technology can be scary or downright frustrating. Remember, using the resources there is a skill, and it does take some practice. If you identify with these statements, try and arrange to use the library with someone who knows their way around and will help you develop your expertise with the processes. Do not allow them to take over, as, although this may be tempting, you have to learn the skills yourself. Do also make use of the library staff. In some libraries it is possible to book a session with a librarian who will show you where everything is and what it does. They should also be happy to help you at any time. Finally, the book by Langford (2001) is written in such a way that is helps the novice to 'navigate the maze' of processes such as using libraries and the Internet. The book, which comes with a CD Rom full of exercises, is a useful way in. Although it is American and focused on nursing in general, it does have sections that relate directly to midwifery and all the skills it covers are transferable.

Extracting relevant details

At the end of the searching phase you should have a reasonable number of references on which to base your review. The next step is to either photocopy, download or order your articles through inter-library loan. Once you physically have your article, it is time to critically assess the material and extract relevant information for your review. To achieve this, you will need to examine all the articles systematically using a critiquing system such as the ones provided in Chapter 5. It is important to state that a review is not written as a series of critiques placed back to back. You need to compare and contrast different studies and comment on the importance of these for the question that forms the aim of the review.

Carnwell and Daly (2001) suggest two useful questions to keep in mind when examining individual papers so that this synthesis can take place later:

Did the methodology of one study produce more valid results than another study?

Does one study have more practical relevance than another study?
(p. 61)

At this stage it is useful to extract information and ideas that can be incorporated into the review. One method favoured by many is to use a fluorescent highlighter pen to mark key passages. Although this is useful as a preliminary stage, it is not useful at the writing of the review stage. This is because they can be over used and you can be left with very few lines on a page that do not have a bright yellow, pink or green line through it! When it comes to writing the review, this is not a useful way of identifying appropriate quotes or points, as they are difficult to locate. The problem of highlighter pens is extended by Langford (2001) who suggests that the use of a highlighter pen when reading encourages lazy thinking. By this she suggests that we need to not only identify relevant information from articles but also think critically about what is said and record some comments of our own.

What are the alternatives to the highlighter pen? One answer is the use of *index cards*. These should follow two systems; firstly, a set of author index cards. Each time an article is photocopied write out a card listing the details using an approved referencing system, or that recommended by the course or institute to which you belong. These cards should be kept in the correct system (either in alphabetical order or the sequence in which they occur in the text). These are useful to check each time you see a new reference as you can easily check whether you already have a copy.

The second system of cards is your *quote cards*; on these you can copy the material highlighted or underlined. These 'quote cards' should also have the name of the author and year of publication to cross-reference with the author cards. They should also include the page number so the quote can be relocated, and the theme under which the quote will be filed (see Figure 6.2).

The last point on writing under theme headings is important, as it allows you to look at the literature as a whole, comparing and contrasting different

P58   Solutions

All maternity services should have an information and support strategy.
As a starting point, local qualitative research is needed to find out what
women want to know and what services could be developed to meet
their needs. Action should be taken to improve women's access to
and use of reliable information and opportunities to talk over issues
during pregnancy.

                                                        Singh et al (2002)

Fig. 6.2   Example of a 'Quote' card

authors under a theme, rather than considering papers individually. As a
guide, reviews are frequently built around the answers to the questions
posed in Box 6.1. Once an appropriate theme is written on a card, those relating to similar themes should be kept together in a suitable small box file with
theme dividers. When it comes to the writing stage, the cards for a particular theme can be spread out so you can clearly see the information gathered
and the issues they cover. Those points that are similar can then be discussed
together by saying such things as 'many authors agree that, etc'. The cards
also allow you to plan the sequence of points planned out before the writing
begins. This is a lot easier than having information underlined throughout
the numerous photocopies you may have, and be faced with the difficulty of
trying to remember what information is where.

   An alternative to index cards is the use of a critique 'grid'. This consists of
a large sheet of paper, such as flip chart paper, or even the back of a sheet of
wallpaper, divided into columns. Each column should contain one of the
theme headings, again using Box 6.1 as a guide, but ending with 'my comments' in which you write any comments that particularly strike you about
the work. Where articles are research, the following columns will also be
useful to act as a summary and allow comparisons to be made between
different articles:

◆   Terms of reference/hypothesis
◆   Research design/method of data collection
◆   Sample size and inclusion and exclusion criteria
◆   Main results (briefly)
◆   Conclusion
◆   Recommendations
◆   Strengths and limitations of the study.

As with the card system, when reading an article or book it is possible to
skim, or speed-read until material relevant to one of the headings in the grid
is encountered. The material is then read slowly and a decision made as to

whether some or all of this should be entered in the grid. You will find it useful to put the page number after each quote you insert in the grid in case you have to relocate it, or need to give the page reference where you use it as a direct quote.

Once an article has been exhausted, a line is ruled across the page and a new article examined. Material relevant to each column will not necessarily appear in each paper, so some columns may be blank for some authors. The advantage of this method is that all material relating to the same theme can be read by looking up and down a column and analyzed for a pattern of similarities or differences between authors, or over time.

A number of reviews of the literature now include sections from such summary tables to summarize sections or themes from the review. These make it easier for the reader to see the bigger picture. It is far easier for the reviewer to refer the reader to a table indicating a key point such as variations in sample size, or type of solution suggested by authors rather than explain complex details in words.

A final method of extracting material relates to the use of a personal computer. If you normally produce your written work directly on a word processing program, the following system will save a lot of time. Instead of using a grid, create a number of files and name each one according to the themes you have decided to use in your review. As you work your way through each source of information, you can open the appropriate file and type in the comments you wish to record. Start each quote with the name of the author, the year of publication and page number. Time can be reduced on a number of word processors if you highlight the author's name and year of publication, and 'copy'. This will then be placed on the computer's 'clipboard'. Each time you add another quote from the same source, use the 'paste' function. The author's name and year of publication will appear ready for you to add the page number and the quote you want to record. You can continue to paste in the name and year for each additional entry, providing nothing further has been copied, as this will 'over-write' what is on the clipboard. If you use this word processing system you may want to print out a hard copy to check the material visually. You can also reorder the material if you so wish.

As all these systems work on the basis of the same principle, you can use whichever one seems most comfortable to you. You can even design your own system, such as the use of a computer spread sheet system instead of the grid system on paper copy. These systems are all designed to make the writing of the review easier by making it easier to locate and manipulate the information taken from the review material.

Common questions

At this stage there are usually a number of questions you may have concerning the review. One of the most frequent question asked by students is *'how many articles do I need for my review?'* Unfortunately, there is no magic number. The advice is to get hold of as many articles as you can in as short a period of time as possible. The more articles you gather, the easier it will be to see a pattern. If time is limited, there should be two main priority areas: include as much recent material as possible, as these will contain current thinking and evidence, and secondly, include as many of the 'classics' as possible. The latter are the titles that seem to appear in the majority of writers' work on a particular topic.

A second question is *'how far back do I need to go?'* The usual method is to go back three or five years. If there is a lot of material, it may be relevant to make the time period shorter such as three years; if there is very little material, it may be beneficial to go back further, such as ten years. However, it is unwise to go further than ten years for material other than classic or seminal work, as changes in health care and social factors mean that information will most likely be difficult to apply to the present.

A further question is *'do all the articles have to be research articles?'* The answer to this is that it is acceptable to include some descriptive reports based on individual thoughts, opinions or experiences, but where possible concentrate on research articles as they are the result of a more systematic process.

A final question is *'can I use what one author says about another author's work?'* This relates to the use of *primary* and *secondary* sources. A primary source is the original work of an author, a secondary source is where someone has quoted, or examined the work of another author. Where it is not possible to get hold of the original work quickly, it is tempting to use secondary sources. These can appear useful where they include critical comment on the primary work. However, although secondary sources are useful to gain a different view on an author's work, LoBiondo-Wood and Haber (2002) emphasize that a credible literature review reflects the use of mainly primary sources.

Writing the review

Writing a critical review of the literature is a high level skill. It is not simply a collection of quotes, 'cut out' of the literature and pasted together, nor is it a series of critiques of individual research articles. It should contain both description of the literature with analysis and reflection on what the literature contains, how well it is presented, and how it all relates to the question the review is seeking to answer. The approach used in writing the review is brought out in the following observation from Benton and Cormack (2000):

> *A review of the literature should be written objectively, with criticism based on factual material and supported by appropriate evidence and argument. In addition, any review should be balanced with both the positive and negative aspects of material being discussed. Furthermore, the implications of any flaws identified in previous work must be highlighted. A good literature review will provide far more than the critical appraisal of a series of articles, it should create a structure upon which further research can be based.*
> (p. 108)

This gives clear guidelines to follow in using the material gathered. The important point is that it should not be the writers' views supported by selected quotes, neither should it be biased by personal preferences. There

1. Decide on a clear question you want to answer through the review.

2. Plan the structure of the review by thinking of the themes that will be applicable. Remember that the following are useful starting points: what, why, when, who, how, problems and solutions or advantages and disadvantages.

3. Decide on the key words you may need for the topic.

4. Identify possible sources of locating references, and journal articles. Explore a library armed with your key words. Consult a database such as CINAHL, MIDIRS, or the Cochrane database. Don't forget to be creative, and use backward chaining; if you find articles look at their references, use colleagues, other students, people in education, and specialists in the topic.

5. If there seems too little material, broaden the topic, if there is too much focus the topic down to one aspect.

6. Decide on a time period (frame) to be covered, initially this could be five years. If there is too little, go back further, where there is too much reduce the number of years. Remember, it might be wise to include the classics (seminal work) in the field.

7. As you locate material, whether it is articles, books or reports, ensure that all the information for a complete reference is written on an author index card.

8. Read through the material with your theme headings in mind. Scan fast until you meet with relevant material and then slow down and decide whether to extract it.

9. Enter the important material onto quote cards, a grid, or straight on to your computer file. Don't forget your own comments on the material.

10. Examine your material for patterns by comparing and contrasting different authors.

11. Write a rough draft under the theme headings. Make sure you have both description (what the various authors say) as well as analysis (how well they say it). Make connections between the material for your reader, and don't forget the purpose of the review. Keep telling the reader why the material included is relevant so they are not left thinking 'so what?'

12. When you are ready for the main draft, write a clear introduction and search process, which includes the purpose of the review, the parameters used to select the material (the source of the material, e.g. British and American, and the time period it covers), and the themes that have been used to group the literature.

13. At the end, make sure you relate the literature to practice. What can we say now based on the literature? The conclusion should comment not only on the subject and what has been learnt, but also on the literature as a body of work itself. Is the available literature comprehensive, or are there gaps? Is the research carried out on the subject of a high standard and rigorous, or does it contain weaknesses?

14. Remember, a review is not an essay that puts forward your views supported selectively by the literature. Neither is it a series of critiques. In writing the review, you should always start from the literature; what does it say?

Box 6.3   The process of reviewing the literature

should be a balance between the differing arguments put forward. The strengths and limitations of different approaches used by authors should also be included, so that there are comments on process (the methods) as well as content. But how can we judge the quality of the review in terms of its usefulness? Again Benton and Cormack (1996) make the following suggestion:

> Unless the literature is analysed in detail and the interrelationships between previous publications identified, the quality of the review will be poor. Inadequate analysis and synthesis of literature results in a review that may only present a series of disjointed paragraphs that echo the findings of previous studies. By planning the review, a logical, structured and coherent argument for further research, or an appraisal of the current state of our knowledge can be presented.
> (p. 109)

The point made here is to avoid the temptation to include as many references as possible, simply because they have been found. They must make sense within the review. The number of references used is much less important than the relevance of the references, the quality of the comments and the overall organization. In the end it must answer the question that has been stated as the aim of the review, and end by saying what we can now say about the topic based on the literature, in particular what is the relevance to practice, or midwifery knowledge.

At this stage it is possible to suggest a systematic process to follow when review of the literature that takes account of all three sections covered so far. This is presented in Box 6.3.

Conducting research

A thorough review of the literature increases the researcher's ability to plan research effectively and efficiently. So much can be learned from the published work of others, both in terms of content – what has already been established, and process – how have others gone about exploring this topic. It is important that the review is comprehensive. The researcher should take advantage of as many sources of information as possible. There should be an emphasis on more recent material as this may provide information about more recent findings, understanding and new approaches. Classic or seminal pieces of published work and reports should also be included.

The researcher should consider the literature critically, and compare and contrast the views and findings of authors. This should be considered in the light of the intended project. In particular, examine concept and operational definitions, and details of data collect tools. The method of data analysis and presentation should also be considered for the way in which they might be models for the present study.

The review of the literature plays a key role in developing the tool of data collection. The main items that have been identified as important in relation to the topic will be included in the tool of data collection. Similarly, where the researcher develops a conceptual framework of the way in which major concepts are linked will arise from the review of the literature. This is not a part of the research process to be dismissed lightly as it is a fundamental building block of the research process, particularly in quantitative research.

Critiquing research

When critiquing a research article, the review of the literature section can provide vital information on what stimulated the researcher's thinking. The design and the nature of the research question will have been influenced by what the researcher discovered in their review. This should be clearly communicated in the report.

Some of the preliminary pointers the reader should consider include the extent of the review – how much literature is included, and how current is it? Is there any work obviously missing? In particular, the reader should consider the extent to which the writer critically reviews the available literature. Do they identify strengths, weaknesses, and particularly gaps in the literature that will be addressed in their study?

The review of the literature should inform the reader and provide a clear rationale for conducting the study. Reading the review should provide an understanding of some of the key issues related to the topic and should also indicate some of the research that has already been undertaken in the area. In some cases the review will also support the theoretical or conceptual framework that has been used in a study. This will link the key concepts together to show how they relate to each other.

Key Points

◆ A review of the literature is a critical analysis of the pertinent published work on a topic.

◆ Carrying out a review has a great deal to offer individual midwives and clinical areas in increasing the standard of evidence-based practice.

◆ Reviewing the literature is a skill that can be developed through the application of the principles outlined in this chapter.

◆ Finding the literature is influenced firstly by the identification of the relevant key words that allow access to the literature through databases.

◆ Spending time in a well-stocked library is essential, but there are a number of other systems available that will also prove useful, such as the use of MIDIRS. It is important to be systematic in the method used to retrieve information from individual books and articles. This chapter has provided several examples of ways of carrying out this process using index cards, summary grids, or word files.

◆ In writing the review the topic should be presented under relevant themes. A review of the literature is not a series of critiques joined together.

◆ If a review is to be relevant to practice, it should include both description and critical analysis.

References

Benton D and Cormack D (2000) Reviewing and evaluating the literature. In: Cormack D (ed.) The Research Process in Nursing (4th edn). Oxford: Blackwell Science.

Carnwell R and Daly W (2001) Strategies for the construction of a critical review of the literature. Nurse Education in Practice 1(2): 57–63.

Hart C (1998) Doing a Literature Review: Releasing the Social Science Research Imagination. London: Sage.

Hek G, Langton H and Blunden G (2000) Systematically searching and reviewing literature. Nurse Researcher 7(3): 40–57.

Langford R (2001) Navigating the Maze of Nursing Research. St. Louis: Mosby.

LoBiondo-Wood G and Haber J (2002). Nursing Research: Methods, Critical Appraisal, and Utilization (5th edn). St Louis: Mosby.

Parahoo K (1997) Nursing Research: Principles, Process and Issues. Houndmills: Macmillan.

Polit D, Beck B and Hungler B (2001) Essentials of Nursing Research: Methods, Appraisal, and Utilization (5th edn). Philadelphia: Lippincott.

Singh D, Newburn M, Smith N and Wiggins M (2002) The information needs of first-time pregnant mothers. British Journal of Midwifery 10(1): 54–58.

CHAPTER SEVEN

The Research Question

Midwifery has no shortage of questions that need to be answered. However, constructing a sound and researchable question is an art that takes practice and the observation of a number of principles. Careful thought is essential as the success of a project is measured against the question it set out to answer. The research question then, is the gateway into the heart of the research process; the researcher must get this stage right as so many other parts of the research process are influenced by it.

But where do research questions come from and what makes a good question? This chapter will outline their importance, and address some of the issues relating to their construction. The purpose of a hypothesis will also be examined, and the different forms they take will be outlined.

The role of the research question

If we compare research to setting out on a journey, then the research question is the statement of the destination. We cannot map a clear and effective route unless we know where we are going, and we certainly will not know whether we have arrived, unless we know where we wanted to be at the end of the journey. In the same way, the research question allows the researcher to plan the research in the best possible way, and make important decisions to ensure that the correct destination is reached.

The following are aspects of the research process that will differ depending on the way in which the research question is phrased:

◆ The broad research approach (methodology)
◆ The tool of data collection (the method)
◆ The sample
◆ The form of data analysis
◆ The ethical considerations.

We can see now what Cormack and Benton (2000) mean when they say:

> Unless you have a clearly defined research question, you will be unable to progress your study in a planned and efficient manner.
> (p. 79)

Research questions evolve from the choice of a particular topic area. This is often a topic felt to be problematic or where questions are raised on what is best practice in relation to providing care. The choice of topic can be prompted by a desire to improve the quality of services, whilst others arise from reviewing the literature, or from searching for ways to provide clinically effective care. All of these can and do lead to someone deciding that the best way forwards is to carry out a research project.

Can research answer every kind of midwifery question? The answer is 'no'. Some questions demand a value judgement for their resolution, and are not open to research. For example, 'should midwives carry out some of the more technological procedures currently performed by obstetricians?' Although we can survey midwives' views or those of obstetricians, the answers would not indicate whether it is 'right', only what people feel about it. Similarly, some questions are ethical or philosophical questions and cannot be answered by research but need to be discussed and debated.

Further light is shed on this issue by Burns and Grove (2001) who propose that questions about practice fall into three categories:

1. Questions answered by existing knowledge
2. Questions answered with problem solving
3. Research generating questions.
   (p. 94)

The first option is important as it illustrates that we should not dash off to do research without checking whether there is already knowledge available to answer our question. That is why we should carry out a review of the literature as a preliminary to research. Their second category relates to the need for debate, reflection and problem solving. The third category is the one in which we are interested.

One important consideration before pursuing a research question is that of relevance. Does the research need to be done? Every project should be evaluated in terms of the contribution it will make to midwifery. This may be in terms of increasing knowledge, or practice, developing or testing midwifery theory, or helping to shape policy. Cormack and Benton (2000) further develop the issue of relevance and suggest the following criteria:

> First does the question address a problem which affects large numbers [of people]? Second, will the outcome of the research significantly improve the quality of life of individuals or groups? Third, does the question address a nursing or midwifery problem? Finally, will the results be suitable for use in a (non-research) practice environment?
> (p. 82)

Perhaps the most important criteria in judging the relevance of a research project is will women, their babies and the family unit stand to gain from this research? Even if the topic relates to midwives themselves, those receiving care may still benefit indirectly through an increase or change in midwives' knowledge, skills or attitudes.

The final point made by Cormack and Benton is also important; unless it is possible to introduce the change into midwifery practice, and overcome the barriers of cost, lack of training or skills, and particularly resistance to change, the research will be a wasted effort.

Having considered the relevance of a particular study, the next major issue is feasibility. This includes such factors as the time available, researcher expertise, ethical consideration, resources available, subject availability and the co-operation of others. The researcher must be able to confirm that all of these issues can be successfully addressed before the research can go any further.

Types of research questions

Research questions are structured in a number of different ways according to the level of question (Brink and Wood 1994) (see Chapter 2). The way the question is written or 'framed' will illustrate the level it addresses. Each level is associated with an appropriate broad research approach. For example, a level one question will suggest the use of a survey or a qualitative approach such as an ethnographic or phenomenological study. Level one questions are those where little is known about a topic and the intention is to describe a situation. There is only one variable in a level one question and one population to which it belongs. The researcher should give a clear concept definition that relates to the way the variable will be defined for the purposes of the study. There should also be an operational definition in a quantitative study that will outline the way it is intended to measure that variable. At this level there is no attempt to establish cause and effect relationships between variables.

A level two question may also suggest a survey, but the question will be concerned with the pattern or correlation between variables. This level may also involve the collection of physiological measurements through observation or taking samples where at least two different measures from each subject are compared statistically to see if they show a similar pattern or correlation. In a level two question more is known about the topic. Here the purpose of the research is to establish if there is a statistical relationship in the form of a correlation between the variables that have been identified. At this level, according to Brink and Wood (1994), although the researcher might have a shrewd idea of what to expect, there is not enough firm evidence from a randomized control trial to confidently predict an outcome and so achieve a level three question.

A level three question will look for a cause and effect relationship between two variables, particularly in relation to a clinical outcome. In a level three question there will be quite a lot known about the nature of the relationship between the variables in the study, enough to make a confident prediction. The purpose is to examine why a relationship exists, or to test a theory. This is achieved by manipulating the dependent variable to measure its effect on the dependent variable in an experimental design study such as a randomized control trial.

Some of the questions midwifery research attempts to answer and how these are related to the level of question are shown in Table 7.1.

Examining the research questions will also suggest a particular method of data collection that might accurately answer the question. Although in many cases a choice may exist, such as the use of questionnaires or interviews, the nature of some questions will suggest which method might be more appropriate. So, if the question is broad, or more abstract, or if it is a delicate or sensitive topic, an exploratory interview will be more appropriate than a questionnaire. Conversely, if the question requires specific and straightforward information, particularly where the likely responses fall into a small number of alternatives, a questionnaire will be a more appropriate method of collecting the data. If the question is about behaviour, then providing it is feasible and acceptable, observation may be more appropriate than depending on memory or the provision of complex details through interviews or questionnaires. A level three question will usually make it clear that a form of experimental design will be needed because it involves decisions on what is more effective, appropriate or successful.

The question will also suggest the type of data to be collected. In the main this will relate to whether quantitative data will be gathered, in the form of numbers, or whether qualitative data in the form of words will be necessary.

Table 7.1   Examples of the type of question, approach, method and data produced

Question	Approach	Method	Data
How much, many, often, what do people think, believe, how well are we doing? (Level 1)	Descriptive quantitative survey, audit.	Observation, questionnaires, interviews, documents	Numeric
What is the lived experience, how do people behave, interpret situations? (Level 1)	Descriptive, qualitative, phenomenological, Ethnographic	In-depth interviews, observation, documentary accounts (diaries, etc.)	Words in the form of dialogue, quotes, observation
Which variable is related to another, or series of others? Does this method correlate with a better outcome than another? (Level 2)	Correlation survey, physiological measurement Quasi experimental	Physiological tests, measurement scales, questionnaires, interviews observation, documents	Numeric
Is this method better than another? Is there a cause and effect relationship between an independent and dependent variable? (Level 3)	Randomized control trial	Physiological tests, measurement scales, questionnaires, interviews observation, documents	Numeric

Constructing a research question

How do we construct a research question? Cormack and Benton (2000) suggest that research questions can occur in one of two forms: the *interrogative* or the *declarative*. The interrogative form is structured in exactly the same way as a question. For example, 'what influences women to continue breastfeeding further than four weeks?' The second declarative form is used more often in research reports, and is a statement of the purpose of the study. This identifies what particular event, phenomenon or situation the study is to consider and usually starts with such statements as:

◆ to examine
◆ to identify
◆ to describe
◆ to explore.

An example would be *'to identify some of the factors that influence a woman to breastfeed further than four weeks'*.

In Chapter 2 we defined this way of expressing the research question as the terms of reference of a study. In other words, this is the statement the researcher 'refers to' in designing the study and collecting the data. The statement of the terms of reference should allow the reader to envisage what will happen to whom. This means there should be an indication of what information is to be gathered, or what variable is being examined, perhaps in relation to another variable, and from whom or what this information will be collected. Table 7.2 illustrates some examples of terms of reference written in this style.

When constructing a research question an easy way to develop the terms of reference is to say 'what is the purpose of my study?' The answer, starting with the word 'to...', will form the terms of reference.

Table 7.2 Examples of terms of reference

Author	Terms of reference	Level
Robinson (2001)	To explore the experience of women who had given birth to a normal baby after screening high-risk for Down's syndrome in the quadruple test. (Qualitative)	1
Bennett et al (2001)	To discover how midwives feel about the public health strategy as outlined in *Making a Difference*. (Quantitative)	1
Jones (2000)	To evaluate the effect and benefit of taught pelvic floor exercises in the prevention of stress incontinence following childbirth. (Correlation)	2
Steen and Marchant (2001)	To evaluate the effectiveness of a new cooling device (gel pad) and compare it with a standard regime (ice pack) and a no localized treatment regimen (control). (Randomized Control Trial)	3

How does the researcher know how to phrase the terms of reference, and which level of question to develop? It is not an easy process, and requires practice and experience. Lo-Biondo Wood and Haber (2002) are at pains to point out that the researcher will spend a great deal of time refining the original idea into a testable research question. The more specific research questions are, the more direction they will provide for the study. Although the researcher may start with a clear statement of the research problem, it is important they examine the literature carefully to establish what is known about the topic. In particular, they should search for possible relationships between the variables in the study. At this stage the researcher should examine the way similar studies have framed their questions, and the way in which they have provided concept definitions and operational definitions for variables as these may be useful in developing a new study.

Lo-Biondo Wood and Haber (2002) suggest the researcher should check that the terms of reference possess the following characteristics:

1. It clearly identifies the variables under consideration
2. It specifies the population being studied
3. It implies the possibility of empirical testing.

The final two points are worth commenting upon. The terms of reference should give some clue as to whom or what the findings will be applied to, and as a consequence, from whom or what the data will be collected. The final point suggests that it should be feasible to collect data to answer the terms of reference, that is, that it is possible to collect the data in the real world.

The hypothesis

In level two and three questions, it is possible to find a hypothesis. This can be defined as the prediction the researcher makes at the beginning of the study that links an independent variable to a dependent variable. As level one questions have only one variable we can see why they do not require a hypothesis. LoBiondo-Wood and Haber (2002) provide the following definition:

Hypotheses can be considered intelligent hunches, guesses or predictions that help researchers seek the solution or answer to the research question.
(p. 52)

The purpose of the hypothesis is to provide a means of demonstrating whether the researcher's prediction can be accepted or rejected. Researchers do not say that a hypothesis has been *proved* or *disproved*, as it is difficult to be that definitive. From the researcher's point of view, a hypothesis gives the study direction, as the design must take into account how the variables will be measured and the statistical way the results will be tested to see if a relationship between the variables can be established. Polit et al (2001) suggest that they force the researcher to think logically and to exercise critical judgement by considering the study within the context of current knowledge and literature.

The hypothesis can take a number of forms, as illustrated below.

Directional/simple

Here a prediction is made as to the likely outcome between two variables, e.g. women who deliver in a midwifery-led unit will have a lower level of intervention during the delivery than those on consultant-led units. Here the dependent variable is the level of intervention, and the independent variable is the form of care. The hypothesis is directional, or one-tailed, because we have predicted the results will be *more than*, or *less than* that found in a comparable situation. A study with this kind of hypothesis could be a level two question where we are comparing midwifery-led care and consultant-led care and looking for correlation between the type of care and level of intervention, or it could be experimental where we randomly allocate women to either a midwifery-led unit or consultant-led unit. In this case it would be a level three question, as we would be deliberately manipulating the independent variable, the form of care and looking for a more explicit cause and effect relationship.

Non-directional

With this kind of hypothesis, although a prediction is made, it is not stated in which direction the outcome will be more favourable, e.g. there will be a difference in the level of intervention in those women who deliver in a midwifery-led unit in comparison with those who deliver in a consultant-led unit. In this example it could be that those delivered in the midwifery-led unit will have less intervention, or vice versa. All that is predicted is that there will be a difference. This form is called a two-tailed hypothesis as the result could go in either of two directions (or tails). A non-directional hypothesis would be used where the researcher feels there is an association, or relationship but is uncertain of the exact nature and so keeps the direction of the findings open.

Null-hypothesis

A null-hypothesis follows the convention in experiments where the researcher demonstrates a lack of bias by stating that they do not expect to find a difference between the two groups in the study, e.g. there will be no difference in the level of intervention at delivery between those women who deliver in a midwifery-led unit or those who delivery in a consultant-led unit. This is also related to statistical convention where if a difference is found, then the null-hypothesis (that there is no difference) has to be rejected. In other words, it has been demonstrated that there is a difference between the groups included in the study. The null-hypothesis is known as the hypothesis of no difference.

The null-hypothesis is known as the *statistical hypothesis* as the aim is to establish statistically whether there is sufficient evidence to accept or reject it. If the statistical hypothesis is rejected then its opposite, the scientific or *research hypothesis* is accepted. The statistical hypothesis and the research hypothesis are different sides of the same coin where in reality one cannot exist without the existence of the other, its opposite. Which one is 'face-up' or currently accepted, depends on the strength of the statistical evidence to support it. The research hypothesis is another name for the first two examples of the hypothesis examined above, that is the directional or non-directional hypothesis.

Not all experimental research states a hypothesis; where they are provided, medical research tend to use the null-hypothesis form and midwifery and nursing research tend to use the research hypothesis suggesting the nature of the outcome.

Complex hypotheses

This form of the hypothesis is very similar to the simple hypothesis except there is more than one dependent variable, e.g. women who deliver in a midwifery-led unit will have a lower level of intervention during the delivery and a lower level of analgesia than those who deliver in a consultant-led unit. It is more usual to see hypotheses expressed separately as two simple hypotheses, as this makes them easy to test and understand.

An example of a complex hypothesis is provided by Steen and Marchant (2001). See if you can identify the dependent variables in the following:

> *The following hypothesis was tested: the use of a new treatment (cooling gel pad) is more effective at reducing levels of perineal pain, oedema and bruising, following either a normal or an instrumental delivery, involving the suturing of an episiotomy or second degree tear, when compared with the standard regimen (ice pack) or no localized treatment (control).*
> (p. 256)

It is more usual to see the dependent variables listed separately in a number of hypotheses as it helps clarity if some are rejected and some are accepted. Here, the dependent variables are perineal pain, oedema and bruising.

Conducting research

For those undertaking research, the development of the research question is one of the most important steps in the research process. The preliminary stages involve ensuring that a problem area does need to be tackled through research. This concerns the relevance of the topic. It is also important to check that the study is feasible in terms of access to the sample; the resources required to carry out the study, the ethical implications, co-operation from key people involved, and the skills of the researcher, as well as the availability of sufficient time to complete the research.

A thorough review of the literature is crucial, as this will provide valuable background information on the topic, including the possible relationships between variables that might have already been discovered. It is also useful for discovering the way other authors have developed concept and operational definitions for the variables. The literature will help the researcher decide on an appropriate level of question. The methods used in previous studies, including the way the data have been analyzed, will also inform the design.

The statement of the research question should be clear. The researcher must be confident that it is possible to answer the research question through data collection. It should make reference to the sample from whom the data will be gathered, and where there is more than one variable, the nature of any relationships should be made clear.

If the level of the question is level two or three, then a hypothesis may be constructed to demonstrate the prediction to be tested through data collection, and whether an association is being considered or a cause and effect relationship.

Once the research question has been constructed, along with the hypothesis if appropriate, it is worth asking, 'will the information I am collecting allow me to answer the terms of reference?'

The final check is to ensure that the research question is not too large to be undertaken in its entirety. Would it be better to take an aspect of this problem area and leave the larger questions either to a future project or to someone else?

Critiquing research

The research question, in the form of the terms of reference, is a key element in critiquing a research article. This is because so many decisions follow as a consequence of the nature of the question. The level of the question, for instance, dictates whether the design should be descriptive or experimental. It is important that the researcher is consistent in the design, which should flow from the question.

The location of the terms of reference is usually in the abstract under the title in those journals that provide one. It is also commonly found just above the subheading 'method' following the review of the literature. Look for the phrase 'the aim of the research was to ...' – the words stating with 'to' will form the terms of reference.

If the question is level two or three, there may be a stated hypothesis, although many researchers appear to omit this. Where a hypothesis is stated, consider whether it is directional, non-directional, or a null-hypothesis. Does it indicate a relationship between an independent and dependent variable in a named sample, and is the nature of that relationship stated? Is the researcher looking for an association, or a cause and effect relationship between the variables? If it is the latter, then the study should be experimental and the researcher should have introduced the independent variable.

Whether we are dealing with one or several variables, in quantitative research the researcher should provide concept and operational definitions for each one identified in the terms of reference or hypotheses. Are these clear and unambiguous?

Finally, at the end of the research article consider whether the researcher has clearly answered the terms of reference? Is there a clear conclusion that relates to and echoes the way the terms of reference were worded? Where the researcher stated one or more hypothesis, is there a clear statement as to whether these have been accepted or rejected? Most importantly, given the results of the research, do you feel the terms of reference have been adequately answered?

Key Points

◆ Research studies revolve around collecting information to answer the terms of reference, or study aim.

◆ The way these are constructed will influence the level of the question and the way the study is constructed.

◆ Research questions must be capable of being answered; they must be feasible and above all relevant.

◆ Level two and three questions may have a stated hypothesis that provides an indication of the prediction the researcher is making between the variables in the study.

◆ Hypotheses come in different forms; they can be simple, complex, directional, non-directional, or a null-hypothesis. Each one has a different purpose and should be used in the right context.

References

Bennett N, Blundell J, Malpass L and Lavender T (2001) Midwives' views on redefining midwifery 2: public health. British Journal of Midwifery 9(12): 743–746.

Brink P and Wood M (1994) Basic Steps in Planning Nursing Research (4th edn). Boston: Jones and Bartlett.

Burns N and Grove S (2001) The Practice of Nursing Research: Conduct, Critique, and Utilization (4th edn). Philadelphia: W.B. Saunders.

Cormack D and Benton D (2000) Reviewing and evaluating the literature. In Cormack D (ed.) The Research Process in Nursing (4th edn). Oxford: Blackwell Science.

Jones M (2000) Pelvic floor exercises: A comparative study. British Journal of Midwifery 8(8): 492–498.

LoBiondo-Wood G and Haber J (2002) Nursing Research: Methods, Critical Appraisal, and Utilization (5th edn). St Louis: Mosby.

Polit D, Beck B and Hungler B (2001) Essentials of Nursing Research: Methods, Appraisal, and Utilization (5th edn). Philadelphia: Lippincott.

Robinson J (2001) Prenatal screening: a retrospective study. British Journal of Midwifery 9(7): 412–417.

Steen M and Marchant P (2001) Alleviating perineal trauma – the APT study. RCM Midwives Journal 4(98): 256–259.

CHAPTER EIGHT

Ethics and Research

Research is not simply about the process of data collection; it is also concerned with the behaviour of the researcher and the manner in which the study is conducted. This has to conform to set standards in the relationship between the researcher and those participating in the research. As with clinical practice, it must illustrate respect and maintain the trust that people have in health professionals and health organizations.

Ethical issues are a particular concern in midwifery research as it involves vulnerable women in pregnancy and labour, and babies who are similarly vulnerable (McHaffie 2000). Both need to be respected, and their safety and privacy safeguarded. Midwives work under the midwifery rules (UKCC 1998), and a professional code of conduct (UKCC 1992), and it is right that midwives are accountable for the way in which they conduct themselves when carrying out research.

But what are ethics and how can they be demonstrated in midwifery research? In this chapter the ethical issues raised by research will be examined. These relate to the protection of basic human rights, and the obligations and responsibilities of the researcher in carrying out research. The main issues covered include informed consent, confidentiality, justice, and an assessment of possible benefits from the research balanced against the possible disadvantages for the individual.

The meaning of ethics

Ethics can be defined as a code of behaviour considered correct. Polit et al (2001) suggest the following definition:

> *A system of moral values that is concerned with the degree to which research procedures adhere to professional, legal, and social obligation to the study participants.*
> (p. 461)

Ethics relate to two groups of people; those carrying out research, who should be aware of their obligations and responsibilities in the way in which they carry out their activities, and the 'researched upon', who have basic human rights that should be protected.

As with ethics generally, those relating to research provide a basis for deciding whether certain behaviour can be regarded as acceptable according to agreed principles and values. There are a number of problems implicit in this, as different people may have conflicting views and values on what is acceptable. To overcome this dilemma, Local Research Ethics Committees (LRECs) were set up at health authority level by the Department of Health in 1991. These have now been gradually replaced since April 2002 with Research Ethics Committees (RECs) who act in the same way (DoH 2001a). The role of these committees is to consider research projects at a planning stage to ensure that they conform to national ethical guidelines and standards.

As medical research has been carried out for far longer and is more frequently conducted than midwifery research, it is not surprising that ethical principles have been developed with medical research very much in mind. This means that ethics committees often use the experimental approach synonymous with the 'scientific' method, as the 'gold standard' against which others are measured.

Is it important for all midwives to know about research ethics? The simple answer is 'yes'. Firstly, they are important in making practice research-based, and the ethical standards of a study are as important as the methodological standards achieved. Research cannot be defended and is not morally safe to implement if it does not conform to ethical principles. It throws into doubt the researcher's honesty and integrity concerning all aspects of the study.

Secondly, knowledge of research ethics may also be crucial if the midwife has to act as advocate for an individual mother, baby and family. This may include situations where someone has become involved in research that is not ethical, or where a request for access to women does not appear to be ethical (Behi and Nolan 1995). The RCN (1998) guidelines on research, which have been adopted by midwifery, also point out that nurses and midwives may be called upon to act as witnesses to ensure that free and informed consent has been given prior to involvement in research. Under these circumstances the midwife should be satisfied that the person concerned has received relevant information to make an informed decision, and is not under any duress or coercion to participate.

It should also be remembered that in recent years there has been a number of high profile 'scandals' concerning babies that have made the headlines. Alder Hey Children's Hospital in 1999 was involved in organ retention and the storage of fetuses, allegedly for research purposes by a pathologist, without parental permission. This has made the public very wary about research in the area of maternity and childcare services. In such situations, if midwives are aware of unethical practices they have a duty to report them.

The RCN (1998) have also pointed out that research is more likely to be designed, completed and used in an ethically sound way if all nurses and midwives understand and have thought through the implications of ethical principles. In other words, if those forming the professional health community are conscious of ethical principles and only accept research that conforms to those principles, then those responsible for generating research are more likely to conform to them. All of these situations emphasize the need for a comprehensive knowledge and understanding of research ethics.

Historical development

It is useful to consider the historical development of our current ethical principles so that we can understand their content and nature. Our present guidelines on research ethics have been influenced by a number of internationally accepted codes on the conduct of research. These were developed following the revelation of a number of scientific experiments on humans that were clearly unethical. Following their revelation, it was agreed that society should be protected from anyone who might carry out research that leads to the death or injury of those taking part. Through a series of refinements the codes outlined in Box 8.1 have influenced present day research practice in medical, nursing and midwifery research.

The Nuremberg code

This was developed in 1947 as a result of the human experimentation carried out by the Nazi regime during World War II. The code consists of ten principles that have been influential in the conduct of research, particularly experimental research, throughout the world. The major principle relates to the necessity of obtaining informed consent from those involved in research. Although the code relates to physical interventions, it also takes account of psychological and emotional harm. One criticism of the code is that it depends on self-regulation by the experimenter.

The declaration of Helsinki

These guidelines for clinical research were developed by the World Medical Assembly at its meeting in Finland in 1964 and updated several times including October 2000 (available at http://www.wma.net). In addition to re-emphasizing the principles of the Nuremberg Code, it developed clauses to protect subjects' human rights. An important distinction made in the declaration was between therapeutic and non-therapeutic research. Therapeutic research relates to situations where the individual may potentially benefit physically from the research, whereas in non-therapeutic research subjects probably will not benefit physically, although others may benefit in the future.

The Belmont report

The Belmont Report of 1978 highlighted what has become the three basic ethical principles of research:

  i. Respect for persons
 ii. Beneficence
iii. Justice.

One of the aims of this report was to develop guidelines on the selection of those included in the research. The report emphasizes the importance of the written consent of subjects, and the obligation of the researcher to assess the possible risk and benefits related to those who take part in the research.

Box 8.1   Major international ethical codes

Nursing and midwifery guidelines

Ethical guidelines for nursing research were developed much later than medical ones. The American Nurses' Association (ANA) developed the first principles in 1968, and these have been updated periodically. These covered not only the basic principles regarding the use of human subjects, but also examined the role of the nurse as researcher and practitioner. In Britain, guidelines were produced by the RCN in 1977 and revised in 1993 and 1998. No separate guidelines exist for midwifery, as it is expected that midwives will follow the nursing guidelines.

Research Ethics Committees (RECs)

In Britain, an important development was the establishment of Local Research Ethics Committees (LRECs) (DoH 1991). This was an attempt to standardize the availability and functioning of ethics committees in both the public and private health sector. LRECs have now been superseded by Research Ethics Committees (RECs). The stated purpose of the REC is to protect the dignity, rights, safety and wellbeing of all actual or potential research participants (DoH 2001a). The report suggests that such committees should be approached for research proposals involving:

a. patients and users of the NHS

b. individuals identified as potential research participants because of their status as relatives or carers of patients and users of the NHS

c. access to data, organs or other bodily material of past and present NHS patients

d. fetal material and IVF involving patients

e. the recently dead in NHS premises

f. the use of, or potential access to, NHS premises or facilities

g. NHS staff – recruited as research participants by virtue of their professional role.
    (p. 7)

The last group may be a surprise, as it is often assumed that research involving staff does not need ethical approval, as it does not involve recipients of health care. It should be remembered, however, that staff also have human rights, and if the research is carried out during 'work' time, it is making use of scarce NHS resources.

An important point to emphasize is that RECs are concerned with research and not audit. If a project is clearly audit, or part of management data gathering, then it does not come under the jurisdiction of the ethics committee. If in any doubt individuals should check with their REC. However, audit should be carried out in an ethical, honest and accurate way.

The recommended membership of RECs is a maximum of 18 members covering a broad range of experience and expertise, so that the scientific, clinical and methodological aspects of a research proposal can be considered.

Both sexes and a wide age range should be represented, with a mixture of 'expert' and 'lay' members. It is recommended that at least one-third of the membership should be lay members who are independent of the NHS. At least half of the lay members should be people who have never been health professionals and who have never been involved in carrying out research involving human participants.

The guidelines issued by the DoH (2001a) state that the appointment of members should be by an open process with vacancies filled following public advertisement and by advertisement via local professional and other networks. This seems to provide an ideal opportunity for midwives to be involved in such committees and currently a number do have a midwife as a member. The DoH document clearly states that those sitting on such committees are not representatives of specialities or departments, but sit as individuals in their own right. This provides even more justification for midwives to understand the principles of research ethics, although the guidelines state that potential members will be given full training.

In America the equivalent of the REC is the Institutional Review Board (IRB). This is required to have at least five members of various backgrounds, who reflect professional, gender, racial and cultural diversity. Membership must include one member whose concerns are non-scientific, such as a lawyer, member of the clergy and at least one member from outside the health organization. The role of the IRB, as with the REC, is to protect those involved in research from undue risk and loss of personal rights and dignity (LoBiondo Wood and Haber 2002).

Ethical principles concerning basic human rights

According to the DoH (2001b) the dignity, rights, safety and well-being of participants must be the primary consideration in any research study. These are highlighted and addressed through ethical principles relating to human rights. In this section the three basic human rights of *respect for individual autonomy*, *protection from harm* and *justice* will be examined within the context of research. In order to clarify the issues, these principles are presented in Table 8.1. This outlines for each of the principles how the researcher demonstrates it has been achieved, and, just as importantly, some of the elements that would suggest that the basic human rights have been denied.

Respect for individual autonomy

This concept is based on the principle that an individual has the right to make free choices about themselves and their life and be 'self-governing', that is autonomous (RCN 1998). This is a familiar concept in midwifery where women are increasingly encouraged through empowerment to be in control of what happens to them (McHaffie 2000). Similarly in research, it is not for us to make people's mind up, or act as though it is not possible to refuse to take part in research.

How is respect for individual autonomy achieved? Table 8.1 illustrates that this principle is demonstrated through the researcher gaining informed

Table 8.1 Issues involved in achieving an ethical study

Basic human principle involved	Achieved through	Denied by
Respect for individual autonomy	Informed consent	Right to refuse to participate or to withdraw at any point not explained. Lack of clear written information on the study given to subjects. Comprehension of information not checked. Confidentiality and anonymity not assured. Coerced to participate. Excessive or unrealistic rewards promised. Deception regarding study details. Existing relationship between researchers and subjects exploited. Covert data collection.
Protection of participants (Beneficence/ non-maleficence)	Risk versus benefit ratio	Risks outweigh benefits. Unacceptable level of pain, discomfort or distress. Confidentiality and anonymity not protected. Access to original data not safeguarded. No debriefing provided or referral to appropriate agencies offered where appropriate.
Justice	Fair selection of sample	Only vulnerable or disadvantaged group included. Captive group used, or coerced, with no opportunity to refuse or withdraw without application of sanctions.

consent from those who take part in a study. The DoH (2001b) suggest that informed consent is at the heart of ethical research. However, this is not a simple matter of gaining approval, or simply agreeing to take part. The important word is *'informed'* consent. For this to be achieved the following elements should be included:

◆ Full disclosure of details about the study
◆ A statement that there is no obligation to take part, and that there are no consequences if the decision to participate is 'no'
◆ Assurance the individual can withdraw at any time without any negative consequences
◆ Confirmation of confidentiality and anonymity
◆ Care that all the information is understood
◆ Provision of an opportunity to ask questions
◆ Absence of pressure, unfair inducements or coercion to take part.

The purpose of the study

The identification of the researcher and their organization

The nature of the participation (what will happen over what period of time)

Possible risks or implications of participating, and any anticipated benefits

Assurance of confidentiality

Informed they need not volunteer

Assured they have the right to withdraw at any time

Offered the opportunity to ask questions.

Box 8.2   Information required to achieve informed consent

What should the researcher tell a prospective subject in a study before we can say that a decision to participate was informed? A good way of thinking about this is to imagine that someone approaches you and asks if you would take part in their research. What information would you want to know before you said 'yes'?

Your answer may be quite a long list including who the people were; what organization they represented; what it will involve, particularly if there is anything invasive, painful, risky or embarrassing; the aim of the project, and what will happen to the information gathered. Anyone participating in research has the right to expect all of these queries to be answered if autonomy is to be protected. The researcher must ensure that all the details included in Box 8.2 are covered before they can claim that informed consent has been sought.

An excellent example of informed consent is provided by the DoH (2001b) in their research governance framework for health and social care guidelines. In box A 'Protecting Research Participants Rights' (p. 9), they provide a scenario between a researcher involved in a study of adopted children and a parent whose child has been approached to take part in the study. This leads on to a discussion between the researcher and the eight-year-old child. This is a very vulnerable and sensitive area that is handled expertly here and provides the ideal guide for any researcher.

The example illustrates that gaining consent is not simply a matter of giving information; the researcher must ensure that the information is given in words that the individual can understand. An attempt must be made to ensure that this has been understood. This relates to the principle of comprehension. In some instances a judgement may have to be made on the competency of the individual to understand the information and the implications of it.

This may also apply to the circumstances under which consent is gained. It is now accepted as undesirable that women be recruited into studies when they are in labour as they are very vulnerable and under other circumstances may not make the same decisions as they might at that time.

In this respect the issue of exploitation must also be considered. This relates to the unfair use of an existing relationship to influence consent to take part in the study. A midwife who has had a long and intimate relationship with a woman may be exploiting that relationship by approaching her to take part in a study. It is very important, therefore, to be able to demonstrate that the consent has been made on a voluntary basis and is free from coercion, or pressure, particularly when people are vulnerable to such approaches. In such circumstances it is better if a third party approaches people for permission.

Consideration has also to be given to gaining written consent. The DoH (2001a) suggest that written consent forms should be included with the application for ethical approval along with simply written information sheets for people explaining the nature of the study.

Confidentiality and anonymity

A vital component of informed consent is the assurance of confidentiality and anonymity. Mander (1995) points out that although these two concepts are often treated as though they are synonymous, they are very different. Confidentiality is a basic ethical principle used in many professional settings, such as the law and the church. Anonymity, Mander points out, is just one of the ways in which confidentiality is maintained. Anonymity means that steps are taken to protect the identity of an individual by neither giving their name when presenting research results, nor including identifying details that might reveal their identity. This might include such things as personal characteristics or the name of work areas where it may be possible to deduce, with reasonable accuracy, the identity of the individual.

Mander (1995) suggests that confidentiality relates to the situation or framework in which information is provided by one person to another, and that the framework should be one of trust where anonymity is assured. Confidentiality does not mean that the information will not be shared with others, as research findings frequently include comments from respondents; the key is that the person cannot be identified, and so remains anonymous.

An important aspect of confidentiality is the application of the Data Protection Act 1998, where if names of individuals are kept on computer, the researcher must conform to the regulations of the Act. This involves the right of the individual to see the information that is kept on them, and their right not to have that information passed on to another party.

Avoiding harm

The second ethical principle is that of avoiding harm. This is discussed in the literature under a number of different headings and can be referred to as the protection of subjects, or *beneficence* and *non-maleficence*. As with professional codes of conduct, the researcher has an obligation to protect the rights and welfare of those involved in research. This means that individuals should not experience any harm as a result of the research. Behi and Nolan (1995) define beneficence as doing good, helping, improving and benefiting the individual, while non-maleficence is avoiding harm to individuals.

Although midwifery researchers are unlikely to set out to inflict harm, it should be acknowledged that some form of harm might be a consequence of participating in a study. For example some procedures are uncomfortable or cause some element of pain. However, this is not likely to be lasting or to cause permanent damage. To some extent all research involves some risks, but in most cases the risk is minimal. This would apply to situations where the anticipated risks are no greater than those commonly encountered in our daily life, or those routinely experienced during physical or psychological tests or procedures. This suggests that we need to assess the type, severity and likelihood of the risks involved in a study. This is what is implied by the term 'risk/benefit analysis', which is the way in which the protection of individuals is demonstrated at the design stage.

The categories of risks that may be encountered in research are physical, psychological or emotional, although Burns and Grove (2001) warn they can also be social and economic. Where midwifery research is concerned with examining the effects of a clinical procedure, such as suturing, care of the perineum, or even something as non-invasive as where the midwife places her hands during the second stage of labour, an assessment must be made of potential discomfort, pain and inconvenience. This must be weighed against the possible benefits involved, in the form of quicker healing, a return to normal functioning or quality of life as a result of the change in procedures.

The difficulty is that at the planning stage it may not be possible to say whether the change in procedure will lead to pain or discomfort, or whether there will be clear benefits as a result of the changes. It is possible, as Firby (1995) has pointed out, that individuals may be exposed to harmful effects or side effects, but the counter problem is that in a situation such as a randomized control trial, certain members of the sample may be denied access to beneficial effects of a new treatment or technique. In this situation the researcher must attempt to calculate the element of risks and benefits in the situation. At any time during the study, if those involved are clearly suffering, or if there is reason to suspect that continuation would result in injury, disability, undue distress or, in extreme circumstances, injury or death, then the researcher has an ethical duty to terminate the study.

It should be clear from the last statement that the protection of the individual from harm applies equally to psychological or emotional distress as well as physical consequences. This can occur not only during research involving clinical intervention, but also in surveys involving questionnaires or interviews. This may also be applied to qualitative research involving interviews or observation. These may entail an element of intrusion, embarrassment or, in some cases, such as describing a negative birth experience or the loss of a baby, a high degree of emotional distress and pain, as well as anxiety and guilt. Under these circumstances the researcher must weigh up the costs to the individual very carefully.

It does not mean that such studies should not be undertaken, as they may benefit others through a greater understanding of the experiences described. However, it does emphasize the need for the researcher to be sensitive to this element of harm. This may include identifying whether, in an individual's own interests, it may be wiser to terminate an interview for example. It also means that individuals should be told beforehand that there might be a possibility of painful memories being confronted in the study. If there is a likelihood of emotional distress, then the researcher must be in a position to counsel the individual, or arrange with counselling agencies to accept referrals should the need arise. It is these kinds of details that RECs would expect to see detailed in the outline of intended research projects.

In designing a study, then, the possible degrees of risk need to be considered. Where this is assessed to be no different from everyday experiences, and of a temporary duration, it would be regarded as being at a minimal level. Burns and Grove (2001) suggest that studies that include questionnaires or interviews usually involve minimal risk or can be seen as a mere inconvenience for the subjects. They go on to suggest that other studies may involve unusual levels of temporary discomfort, where subjects experience discomfort both during the study and after it has been completed. For example, an individual may be left feeling physically sore or in pain for some time later. Some qualitative studies may also have similar consequences where individuals are asked questions that involve reliving traumatic experiences or events. Robinson (1996) has suggested that extremely invasive and unreasonably painful questioning can be thought of as 'mind rape'. Although we may feel that this is unlikely to happen within midwifery research, it is essential that we are sensitive to the possibility of respondents experiencing research in these terms.

Suggestions for avoiding psychological harm in interviews have been made by Polit et al (2001). Their recommendations include the tactful phrasing of questions, and the provision of debriefing sessions after an interview to permit participants to ask questions or air complaints. In some situations, they suggest the researcher may need to make a referral to appropriate health, social, or psychological services.

Finally, in terms of the extent of harm, it is possible that some studies could be assessed as having no anticipated elements of harm or benefits for the individual (Burns and Grove 2001). An example would be the collection of information from records or other documents where the researcher is not in direct contact with individuals and where there is no breaking of confidentiality. Audit would fit this category as well as other studies involving records.

Justice

Justice, the third and final human principle, is rarely considered. This relates to the fair treatment of those in the study. In selecting the study population, the researcher should be careful to avoid leaving themselves open to the criticism that only those people who are vulnerable to coercion or suggestion have been included. Providing they do not form a bias, all groups should stand an equal chance of being included in research projects, and should not be excluded because it is considered they have a special privileged status.

This element of justice can be clarified by the following useful list that Polit et al (2001) suggest make explicit the application of fair treatment:

◆   The fair and non-discriminatory selection of participants such that any risks or benefits will be equitably shared; selection should be based on research requirements and not on the vulnerability or compromised position of certain people

◆   The non-prejudicial treatment of people who decline to participate or who withdraw from the study after agreeing to participate

◆   The honouring of all agreements between the researcher and the participant, including adherence to the procedure as described in advance and the payment of any promised financial rewards

◆   Participants' access to research personnel at any point in the study to clarify information

◆   Participants' access to appropriate professional assistance if there is physical or psychological damage

◆   Debriefing, if necessary, to divulge information withheld before the study or to clarify issues that arose during the study

◆   Sensitivity and respect for the beliefs, habits, and lifestyles of people from different cultures

◆   Courteous and tactful treatment at all times.

Problems in research

Firby (1995) has pointed out that as with any ethical dilemma, individuals hold differing moral views and what may seem moral to one person may not be to another. In this section some of the frequently encountered problem areas, or contentious issues will be presented so that the reader can be aware of the problems.

One contentious area relates to informed consent. Part of respecting the individual is to ensure that the purpose of the research is made clear so that the individual is in a position to truly give informed consent. But are there occasions where it is not possible to give complete details of the study without compromising the validity of the results? There are situations where comprehensive descriptions of the purpose of the study will influence the expectations or behaviour of the participants. For example, a study of student midwives' hand-washing techniques may not be accurate if the students are told that hand washing is being observed. To gain more valid results, the researcher may have to say that they are observing routine procedures, and not draw attention to the importance of hand washing. The argument for this kind of incomplete disclosure would have to be made in the application to the REC. However, this situation is not that dissimilar from double-blind studies, where neither the researcher nor the patient knows who is receiving the experimental variable.

Another problem area for the researcher is that of confidentiality. We tend to think of confidentiality as not sharing information. Clearly the purpose of research is to communicate and publish the results, but in a way that will not identify or harm the individual. However, at the point of data collection there are instances where it is not possible to keep confidences, even where they are promised. One example of this is where there is a greater obligation on the midwife researcher to inform others of information that has been given in confidence. Clearly where a respondent in an interview provides evidence of child abuse, the midwife researcher would have to state that the information could not be kept confidential. The first form of action would be to encourage the respondent to report the matter, or to give permission for the researcher to report it. If these options were declined, the midwife researcher would have to report the information. The same would apply to interviews, or observation of staff that involved unsafe or unethical practices. Again the matter would have to be reported.

Cerinus (2001) illustrates that where the researcher provides assurances of confidentiality, the participant may call upon them to support it. This means that what follows may have to be excluded from the study. Alternatively, the researcher may have to break that confidence to report issues related to codes of conduct. Cerinus (2001) quotes examples of how those in her study would preface such incidents with phrases such as: *'Confidentially speaking of course …'*, *'Just between you and me …'* or *'Within these four walls only …'* (p. 81).

This led to Cerinus having to decide whether to break the flow of the interview to remind them of her ethical duty, or wait until later to reassess the situation. In most cases, problems can be solved relatively easily; it is only where matters of professional conduct are concerned that there can be an apparent conflict between the role of researcher and that of midwife. Where the safety of a woman or her baby is concerned, the first responsibility is to their welfare and the demands of research must come second.

In the past a documented problem area has been the actions and decisions of ethics committees who have not always understood or been sympathetic to research proposals from midwives. This particularly applies to undertaking qualitative studies. Some of the problem stems from the power and influence of doctors on such committees and their traditional narrow focus on experimental research. At a recent conference where I presented a paper on the differences between quantitative and qualitative research, I was asked by a member of an ethics committee why qualitative researchers always submitted weak proposals. He complained that the research question was always very vague and no clear details were given of the tool of data collection. In addition the doctor posing the question asked me to agree that the clear lack of any identified improved clinical outcomes meant that such studies were ethically unsound!

The lack of familiarity of such committees with qualitative research approaches is also clearly illustrated by Hunt (Hunt and Symonds 1995) who wished to undertake an ethnographic study involving non-participant observations and informal interviews over a considerable time period. The comments from the doctors on the ethics committee show a complete lack of understanding of the conventions and approach of this type of research, despite a clear explanation provided by Hunt. She describes how she was criticized by one doctor because 'details of the questionnaire to be used were not included', another requested clarification on the control group to be used, and another wanted more details of the statistical tests that would be used. All of these are inappropriate in ethnographic research and had been clearly indicated as such in the proposal.

The standard submission form used by some ethics committees underlines their difficulty in understanding wider approaches to research. The novice researcher can be perturbed by all the references in these forms to what appear to be assumptions regarding the involvement of invasive procedures, drug company sponsors, and the need for specific indemnity cover. The most appropriate solution is to indicate 'not applicable', and if in any doubt to seek guidance from the chair or secretary of the committee. It is hoped that as more midwives undertake research, and become members of RECs themselves, that these problems may diminish.

Conducting research

This chapter has identified the main areas to consider when planning research. All researchers are required to carry out research that reaches agreed standards of ethical conduct, and it is right and proper that they do. The most important principles to address are those of:

◆ Informed consent
◆ Assessment of risk/benefit ratio
◆ Confidentiality of material and anonymity of participants
◆ Fair selection and treatment of subjects.

At the planning stage it is important to discover the whole processes involved in gaining research approval in your clinical area. This can be quite a long chain of events, part of which will be approval by an REC. Once the preliminary stages have been negotiated, contact the secretary of the REC for the appropriate form. This may be supplied in the form of a computer disk. A great deal of thought needs to go into completing this. Ensure that it illustrates that ethical principles have been identified and addressed, and that the approach and methods of data collection have credibility. This can be illustrated by reference to their use in other similar published studies. The tool of data collection should be included in the proposal.

It must be clear that written informed consent will be gained, and that details of the study will be given in writing to those taking part. This will include a clear statement that there is no requirement to participate in the study, and that it is done on a voluntary basis. It should also be clear that the individual can withdraw at any point without feeling that this will affect care.

Both the consent form and study information sheet should be written in plain language and included with the proposal to the REC. Where the tool of data collection is a questionnaire, it can be accepted that a response is an agreement to participate, providing a covering letter has made it clear that participation is voluntary and the nature of the study explained.

The submission to the ethics committee should demonstrate the importance of the study and illustrate that the findings would make a contribution to the service. Careful use of the available literature, and details of the local situation should be used to support these claims.

Where the applicant is new to research, it is expected that a supervisor with research experience will be named. This might be someone within midwifery education, or with previous research experience. Similarly, where the study will entail statistical analysis, the names of those providing statistical advice and support will be required to provide assurance on the accuracy of the results.

Details on how confidentiality and anonymity will be maintained should be included. If names of subjects are not required, do not ask for them. Information on the arrangements for secure data storage should be outlined. It is also wise to state that original forms, or taped interviews will be destroyed or erased once the final report has been accepted.

Finally, it is important to assure the committee that the researcher will not raise expectations that the study will result in the provision of additional services or facilities for those who take part.

Before submitting a proposal to an REC, it is worth discussing the proposal, particularly the ethics sections, very carefully with someone who can give advice on the subject. This may include someone who has had experience of submitting a proposal to that committee.

Even if an REC is not involved or relevant, support from managers will be required. It is always wise to insist on written confirmation of support. Permission to start a study is one of the most important steps in the research process. There can be considerable delays and disappointment if this does not go smoothly. Do everything you can to ensure that the ethical and methodological sections of your research proposal illustrate a high standard, and that these are based on sound knowledge.

It is worth closing this section with the words of Robinson (1996) who warns those about to embark on research that badly designed research is per se unethical and should not be done at all. At best it wastes participants' time and at worst it can do outright harm.

Critiquing research

Although an author may mention some ethical issues in a report, there is not always space to cover all the aspects covered in this chapter. This means that only brief mention may be made of the approval by an ethics committee; the gaining of informed consent, and the assurances of confidentiality or anonymity. Often the reader is left to assume that things have been carefully thought out, and ethical safeguards applied.

It is reasonable for the reader to ask the following questions as a minimum:

◆ Was the study submitted to an ethics committee (REC)? In the case of an American study, is there mention of an Institutional Review Board (IRB)?

◆ Is there evidence of freedom from bias in the way the researcher conducted the study? In particular, did any body or organization that might have had a vested interest in a positive outcome sponsor the author(s)?

♦ Was informed consent gained?

♦ Were there any risks of discomfort or distress involved in taking part in the study not anticipated by the researcher, or not justified by the likely benefits to the individual/others in a similar situation?

♦ Did the researcher conduct the research in a sensitive manner in regard to the wording of questions and privacy afforded individuals?

♦ Were any foreseeable discomforts, side effects or potential risks outlined to subjects before they gave informed consent?

♦ Was a pilot study undertaken that may have identified any risks to the individual?

Key Points

♦ Research is not simply a process of gathering data, but involves ethical considerations in conducting the study.

♦ Ethics relate to the protection of the human rights of those involved in research, and the obligations and responsibilities of the researcher. The main human rights the researcher must consider are respect for the individual, the protection against harm, and justice.

♦ Informed consent relates to the extent to which an individual agrees to take part in a study on the basis of a clear understanding of the purpose of the research and the implications of agreeing to take part.

♦ The 'harm versus benefits' ratio is an attempt to weigh up the possible disadvantages for an individual taking part in a study, against the possible positive effects either for them or others in the future.

♦ Justice relates to the fair treatment of all those who are potentially or actually involved in the research process.

♦ Each area has a research ethics committee (REC) whose role is to examine research proposals so that they can protect the public and health staff against harm and exploitation.

♦ Projects that can be classified as audit usually are not required to be assessed by an ethics committee, but the researcher should still be mindful of the way the information is collected and the use to which it is put.

References

Behi R and Nolan M (1995) Ethical issues in research. British Journal of Nursing 4(12): 712–16.

Burns N and Grove S (2001) The Practice of Nursing Research: Conduct, Critique, and Utilization (4th edn). Philadelphia: W.B. Saunders.

Cerinus M (2001) The ethics of research. Nurse Researcher 8(3): 72–89.

Department of Health (1991) Local Research Ethics Committees. London: HMSO.

Department of Health (2001a) Governance Arrangements for NHS Research Ethics Committees. http://www.doh.gov.uk/research/rd1/researchgovernance/corec.htm

Department of Health (2001b) Research Governance Framework for Health and Social Care. http://www.doh.gov.uk/research/rd1/researchgovernance/corec.htm

Firby P (1995) Critiquing the ethical aspects of a study. Nurse Researcher 3(1): 35–42.

Hunt S and Symonds A (1995) The Social Meaning of Midwifery. Houndmills: Macmillan.

LoBiondo-Wood G and Haber J (2002). Nursing Research: Methods, Critical Appraisal, and Utilization (5th edn). St Louis: Mosby.

Mander R (1995) Practising and preaching: confidentiality, anonymity and the researcher. British Journal of Midwifery 3(5): 289–95.

McHaffie H (2000) Ethics and good practice. In: Proctor S and Renfrew M (eds.) Linking Research and Practice in Midwifery: A Guide to Evidence-Based Practice. Edinburgh: Baillière Tindall.

Polit D, Beck B and Hungler B (2001). Essentials of Nursing Research: Methods, Appraisal, and Utilization (5th edn). Philadelphia: Lippincott.

Robinson J (1996) 'It's only a questionnaire' … ethics in social science research. British Journal of Midwifery 4(1): 41–44.

Royal College of Nursing (1998) Research Ethics: Guidance For Nurses Involved In Research Or Any Investigative Project Involving Human Subjects. London: RCN.

UKCC (1992) Code of Professional Conduct. London: UKCC.

UKCC (1998) Midwives Rules and Code of Practice. London: UKCC.

CHAPTER NINE

Surveys

Gathering data for research is exciting. However, its success depends largely on the method used. This must be appropriate to the research question, and should be a reasonable choice for the sample group. In this chapter we examine the use of the survey, which has traditionally been a popular method of collecting research information from people. A survey can be defined as a way of gathering data by directly asking respondents for information either in the form of a questionnaire or interview.

In the following sections we will examine some of the principles involved in the use of surveys, and then look at the advantages and disadvantages of one method; the use of questionnaires. The principles of questionnaire design will be illustrated at the end of the chapter. The next chapter will examine the use of interviews.

The survey

The survey has become one of the most frequently used methods in the social sciences, and in health care research forms the largest category of non-experimental designs (LoBiondo-Wood and Haber 2002). Midwifery researchers have also found that this method of collecting data ideally suits many of the questions they wish to answer.

Why are surveys so popular? One reason is that they are very user-friendly. They are less intimidating for both the researcher and the subjects of the research in comparison to some of the other forms of data collection. They are also a very economic way of collecting a large amount of data, illustrating the very practical reasons for their popularity.

They are also an incredibly useful way of filling in gaps in our knowledge, as the number of results from surveys announced in the media every day testifies. Polit et al (2001) illustrates this usefulness by saying:

> Survey research is highly flexible; it can be applied to many populations, it can focus on a wide range of topics, and its information can be used for many purposes.
> (p. 186)

In other words, surveys are commonly accepted as a legitimate foundation for decision making in society. Their use has always been a feature of assessing maternity services both by health professionals and consumer groups. This pattern is likely to increase in all areas of health care with the importance placed on user involvement under clinical governance.

The basic principle on which surveys are based is that if you want to know what is going on, then the best way to find out is to ask people. The results can be quantitative in the form of numbers, or qualitative in the form of words.

Surveys can vary in a number of ways, one of the most important being the degree of structure they contain. Very structured surveys are useful if the researcher wants to check the kind of pattern involved with a certain type of activity, such as the number of women who intend to breastfeed, or the information needs of first-time pregnant mothers (Singh et al 2002). This type of survey has the great advantage that the results are reasonably easy to analyze as it frequently involves counting the number who said 'yes' or 'no'. This method is now becoming increasingly used as the basis for audit, where repeated measures of routine information are collected.

However, the disadvantage of this method, as Polit et al (2001) observe, is that it can be a little too superficial. More in-depth information can be gathered using a less structured data-collection tool. However, the researcher can be faced with information overload, and the answers may be very different from each other, making comparisons and summaries difficult.

The survey can vary in relation to the time-period it examines. It can take the form of a 'one-off' collection of data. This is sometimes referred to as a 'cross-sectional' study. Here the intention is to consider how a range of people feel about a subject, or to identify their experiences in relation to a specific event or experience. It is possible to repeat data collection after a period of time with a different group of people to see if there has been a change. The number of women wanting a home delivery could be gathered at one point in time, and then repeated one or more years later to see if there has been a change. This is known as a *trend survey*, and works in the same way as audit where the same measurement is used at different times on different people to see if things have changed.

Longitudinal studies can follow the same group of people over time and keep going back to them to note any changes. This is sometimes called a *panel design* where the researcher goes back to the same group of people over time (Burns and Grove 2001). For instance, Lavender et al (2000) followed women through pregnancy from booking clinic to cover a total of five time points ending with their discharge from midwifery care 14–28 days after the birth. Questionnaires were used at each point to answer the question 'how do women feel about the information currently provided on pregnancy, labour and parenthood?' The aim was to explore issues surrounding the amount, timing, content and format of current information provided to first-time mothers.

There are two problem areas concerning the use of surveys; the first relates to the representativeness of the sample on whom the results are based, and the second, relates to validity, or what is actually being measured. The issue relating to the sample is important as the researcher frequently wishes to generalize the findings to similar people in the wider population. For this reason surveys must try to avoid bias in the way the sample is chosen. The alternative methods of sampling will be covered in Chapter 14.

In designing the survey, it is usual to collect some basic 'demographic' details such as age, staff grade, sex, or number of children, so that some comparison can be made with those in the wider population to see if they are similar. This then gives some indication of how far the sample is representative. The second question of ensuring validity is a difficult issue. One of the problems in surveys is that of the 'words/deeds dilemma' (Couchman and Dawson 1995). This means that what people say is not necessarily what they do. There has to be an element of trust in what people say, as the researcher cannot always test the truth. People may be inclined to give socially acceptable answers in surveys, and so the accuracy can never be 100%. The only action the researcher can take is to try and reduce the amount of distortion produced by the data-collection tool. The pilot study is one method by which this can be attempted.

The use of questionnaires

Questionnaires are probably the most familiar data-collection tool in nursing and midwifery research. Most of us are likely to have received and probably completed at least one questionnaire in our working lives, and perhaps thrown many more away. In this section we will examine some of the advantages and disadvantages of this method and outline some of the important principles of questionnaire design.

A large number of research questions in midwifery have been answered by questionnaire. Why are they such a popular method of collecting research data? Box 9.1 suggests some of the answers.

Although this list suggests that questionnaires are an ideal data collection method, several factors may discourage a response, as Box 9.2 suggests. There are a balancing number of disadvantages to the use of questionnaires. People have now received so many questionnaires that their motivation to complete and return yet another may not be high. For a number of reasons, the proportion returning a questionnaire can be low. If the response rate is below 50%, then there is no certainty that the responses represent the views of those sent one. In other words, we may end up with a biased response. Generalizations from this group would then be impossible. Reminders can be sent to increase the final response rate, although the return from this may also be disappointingly low.

- ◆ Cheap
- ◆ Quick
- ◆ Can reach a large geographically spread sample
- ◆ Can be quite detailed
- ◆ Low level of embarrassment or threat to both researcher and respondent
- ◆ Anonymity is protected
- ◆ Fixed choice questions easy to answer and to analyze
- ◆ Familiar method to respondents.

Box 9.1   Advantages of questionnaires

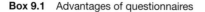

- ◆ Questionnaires have now saturated the population
- ◆ Response rate may be low dependent on feelings on the topic
- ◆ Questionnaires are dependent on literacy and physical ability
- ◆ Responses will be influenced by the quality of the design
- ◆ There is no opportunity for clarification of questions or answers
- ◆ Fixed-choice questions may not have an appropriate alternative for everyone.

Box 9.2   Disadvantages of questionnaires

One important assumption underlying the use of a questionnaire is that recipients can read and write in English. This is not simply an issue of literacy; many people have trouble with eyesight or problems with the ability to write because of physical problems. For this reason we have to remember that surveys involving the public as a whole can miss out important opinions because of certain groups who are excluded because of the choice of method.

The disadvantages of questionnaires relate to both the researcher and the respondent. A recurring frustration for the researcher is receiving returned questionnaires containing a number of unanswered questions, or where they are incomplete in some way. Once returned, it is not possible to clarify answers or probe further. From the respondent's point of view, one irritating feature of questionnaires is to be asked to choose from a range of alternative options where none apply. This raises questions of validity where a respondent is not truly describing their own views or experiences but merely choosing something the researcher has selected.

Holloway and Fullbrook (2001) have also commented that even when open-ended questions are used in questionnaires, they tend to direct and control the respondent in the way in which they answer a question. Bias can also be created, they point out, through the researcher's use of value-laden or leading words. This involves sentences that include words such as 'unnecessary', 'painful', 'appropriate' 'too long', etc., instead of phrasing questions in a neutral way. The conclusion is that as a method the questionnaire has a number of advantages and disadvantages. They are certainly not an easy option to use in research, and have a number of restrictions and limitations. Their success depends on their design as this will influence whether an individual will complete them or not. This is emphasized by Coombes (2001) who suggests that:

> A good questionnaire is not just a list of questions. It will have been carefully planned, drafted and piloted with a few colleagues, have taken into account the likely respondents and throughout the whole process the eventual method of data analysis will have been borne in mind.
> (p. 123)

The message here is clearly do not underestimate the subtlety and skill required in the use of this form of data collection. For this reason the next section will consider some of the principles involved in questionnaire design.

Questionnaire design

The first stage in designing a questionnaire is to ensure that it is an appropriate method for collecting the data. Careful consideration should be given to the advantages and disadvantages outlined above. The terms of reference should also provide some clue as to whether it is appropriate. If this includes mention of finding out what people say or do, or relates to areas where it seems that individuals themselves are in the best position to accurately supply the information, then questionnaires would seem a reasonable alternative. The review of the literature should help to establish whether previous studies have used a questionnaire, and with what success. Once a firm decision has been made to use a questionnaire then the researcher moves into the design stage.

As Murphy-Black (2000) observes, there is much to learn about questionnaire design. It is not simply concerned with writing possible questions. There are three interrelated parts to any questionnaire and each need to be constructed very carefully. These have been identified by Sarantakos (1994) as:

1. The covering letter
2. The instructions
3. The main body.

The covering letter

Before respondents consider answering questions they need some explanation and encouragement to take part in the research. The covering letter plays a crucial role in encouraging the recipients to return the questionnaire. Murphy-Black (2000) observes that the covering letter is vital as it makes the first impression on the respondent, either good or bad. The letter should be persuasive but honest, and should contain some of the elements outlined in Box 9.3.

Instructions

The questionnaire should start with a clear title that summarizes the purpose of the survey and should include a section marked 'Instructions'. This should

---

◆ Who you are and the capacity in which you are writing (e.g. student, member of a clinical team, or manager)
◆ The aim of the study, in broad terms
◆ The reason why the person has been included in the study
◆ Motivation to return the questionnaire (how they, or others, will benefit from completing it)
◆ Assurance on confidentiality and anonymity
◆ Estimate of the time is should take to complete
◆ Contact address/telephone number should they want further details or assurances.

Box 9.3 Elements that should be included in a covering letter

simply and unambiguously tell the respondent the different ways they may be asked to respond to questions. As the respondent works their way through the questionnaire they should be in no doubt as to whether they should tick a box, circle a number or add a comment of their own. The pilot study should provide the opportunity to test the clarity of the instructions, as unless these are successful, valuable data may be lost.

The main body of the questionnaire

The crucial part of the questionnaire is the body of questions. Here we must ensure that there is as little possibility for misunderstanding or inaccuracy as possible. The respondent should find it interesting and easy to complete, and the researcher should find that the replies provide an answer to the terms of reference. If this is to be achieved then thought has to be given to:

1. Choice of questions
2. Wording and structure of the questions
3. Method of answering
4. Analysis of the responses.

The choice of questions

The choice of the questions will be influenced by the terms of reference and the thinking that lies behind it. Where the researcher believes that a number of variables such as parity, previous experience and attitudes towards childbirth influence a situation, these should be included in the questions. The review of the literature will also provide some pointers to relevant questions.

At the design stage there is frequently a temptation to include too many questions. The longer the questionnaire, the less likely it is to be returned. Every question should be relevant to the aim of the research. It is worth the researcher asking 'why am I including this question?' If a clear answer cannot be given, the question should be deleted. It is also an advantage to ask colleagues, and particularly 'experts' in the field, for their view on the choice of topic areas and questions.

The wording and structure of the questions

The wording and structure of the questions need special attention. First, Box 9.4 outlines some of the basic principles of questionnaire design and although these seem straightforward, they are frequently ignored. One valuable piece of advice in questionnaire design is to put yourself in the place of the person completing it; will it make sense to them? Are there certain assumptions being made about the person's knowledge that may not be justified? In following this advice it may be possible to avoid mistakes such as asking questions that are not answerable. An example would be 'do you think the birth of your baby would have been better in a different hospital?' Not only does this give no indication as to what might count as 'better', it is clearly difficult for

- ◆ Give clear instructions on how to complete the questionnaire
- ◆ Give assurances on confidentiality and only ask for name and identifying characteristics (e.g. clinical area if staff) if necessary
- ◆ Questions should relate to the terms of reference
- ◆ Avoid long questionnaires; keep them to 2 to 3 sides
- ◆ Avoid long questions; respondents will lose track of its purpose
- ◆ Avoid a single question asking more than one thing at the same time; split them into separate questions
- ◆ Use simple language and avoid unnecessary or unexplained jargon and abbreviations
- ◆ Use a clear layout to make it attractive on the page, and allow realistic space for written comments
- ◆ Group questions on the same topic together to form a logical sequence
- ◆ Avoid ambiguous questions and vague words such as 'regularly'
- ◆ Avoid leading questions and value-loaded words
- ◆ Avoid presuming that people do things, ask filter questions first
- ◆ Avoid questions with 'no', 'not', 'never' in the question where the alternative answers are 'yes', or 'no' as it can lead to confusion
- ◆ Ensure with fixed choice questions that there is an alternative for everyone, such as 'not applicable', 'don't know' or 'other'
- ◆ If people are unlikely to say 'yes' or 'no' to a question owing to social desirability then the question is not worth including
- ◆ Use Likert scales ('strongly agree', etc. 'often', 'sometimes', 'rarely', 'never') where the answer may not be simply 'yes' or 'no'
- ◆ Include a balance between open and closed questions to avoid repetitiveness
- ◆ Leave sensitive, potentially embarrassing or intrusive questions to later in the questionnaire
- ◆ At the design stage think how you will analyze each question
- ◆ Get comments on your draft questionnaire from colleagues and pilot it before using it to ensure it works (this should include analysis).

Box 9.4 Basic principles in questionnaire design

someone to evaluate whether there would have been differences if the birth had taken place in a different unit.

Vague words are a further problem in the wording of questions. There is a need for clarity of thought that should lead to precision in the wording of questions. Words such as 'regularly' should be avoided as in 'since the birth of your baby are you able to go out regularly?' This does not explain the context in which 'going out' is placed. Does it mean shopping, visiting people or social activities? Nor would it be meaningful as a 'yes' or 'no' response, as 'regularly' could mean vastly different things to different people.

As can be seen from the list of principles in Box 9.4, simplicity is one of the keys to questionnaire design. It is important to use simple words, and avoid jargon or technical terms such as 'primiparae' and 'multiparae' to non staff.

Questions should be simple and short and avoid asking more than one question in a single sentence such as:

Have you more than one child and were any of these born at home?

❑ YES   ❑ NO

This should be divided into two; first it should ask 'have you more than one child and then as a further sub-question: 'If 'yes', were any of these born at home?' This would then appear as follows:

5 a) *Have you more than one child?*   ❑ YES   ❑ NO

   b) *If yes, were any of these born at home?*   ❑ YES   ❑ NO

It is also important to avoid biasing the individual's response with leading questions or emotive words that suggest the appropriate answer, e.g.

Would you agree that the midwife kept you fully informed during the labour?

Would it be more convenient for you to attend antenatal classes in a health centre near your home rather than in hospital?

This last question would be better asked in a more neutral way such as:

If you had a choice of where you could attend antenatal classes? Would you choose:

a) ❑ *Those at my local hospital*

b) ❑ *Those at my local health centre*

c) ❑ *Either one would be acceptable*

The method of answering questions

The method of answering questions can take a number of forms. The example above is called multiple-choice questions where the respondent chooses one of the alternatives offered. This falls into the category of closed questions as opposed to open questions. In open questions the respondent is not offered alternatives to choose from, but is left to express the answer in their own words. An example of an open question would be the following:

What did you hope to gain from attending antenatal classes?

Open questions work well where respondents are used to expressing themselves in writing. They will not work well or be productive with everyone.

Open and closed questions have their advantages and disadvantages. For instance, although closed questions have the advantage of simplicity, they may influence the respondent by suggesting answers that they may not have thought of without the prompt of the fixed-choice alternatives. The open question has the advantage of the respondent using terms and options that they feel describe their own experiences or views, rather than using those offered by the researcher. The disadvantage of open questions is the large amount of data that has to be analyzed and coded before any kind of summary or identification of issues takes place. The ideal compromise is to have a mix of open and closed questions, which maximizes the advantages of both forms of question.

One method of increasing the sensitivity of closed questions is the use of a range of scaling techniques (Burns and Grove 2001). Although we often think of closed questions as having a yes or no answer, where attitude or opinion is concerned, how people feel about an issue or statement may lie anywhere along a continuum. This can be dealt with using a Likert scale, which is named after the American Rensis Likert, who first introduced them. These can take three forms and relate to:

♦ Agreement
♦ Evaluation
♦ Frequency.

In the case of agreement scales, statements in a broad mix of positive or negative forms are given and the respondent is asked to make a choice between five alternatives ranging from strongly agree to strongly disagree. Furber (2000), in her study of midwives' attitudes to health promotion used this approach, and her results section clearly illustrates the use of these categories. Fictional examples are shown below:

i) Agreement
I feel that pain relief in labour should be taken as a last resort
❑ strongly agree ❑ agree ❑ undecided ❑ disagree ❑ strongly disagree

ii) Evaluation
The information I received from the midwife about the alternative forms of pain relief was
❑ excellent ❑ very good ❑ undecided ❑ poor ❑ very poor

iii) Frequency
I get feelings of panic when I think about looking after the baby
❑ always ❑ sometimes ❑ rarely ❑ never

In the last example four choices have been used, as these seem to cover the main alternatives. The inclusion of 'never' removes the necessity to include a neutral mid-category. Some people argue that with example i) and ii) above, the mid-category of 'undecided' should be removed to prevent people choosing a neutral option and sitting on the fence. From experience, this has never been seen in practice. It should also be remembered that there must be an alternative that applies to everyone. There are occasions when a mid-category could be a legitimate choice and should be respected.

The statements or 'items' in the Likert scale should be a mix of those expressed positively and those expressed negatively to prevent respondents simply putting a tick in the same column each time without really thinking about the question. So for instance, the following two examples may be used in a satisfaction questionnaire.

The midwife was too busy to answer my questions

(negative item)

I felt confident with the midwife who conducted the delivery

(positive item)

The order of these statements should not follow a set pattern, for instance, alternately positive and negative; providing there is an equal number of each kind of statement they should be presented in a random order.

A similar technique to the Likert scale is to use a visual analogue scale (VAS) which is a line drawn across the page, usually ten centimetres, with opposite words at each end. The respondent is asked to place a cross on the line to correspond with how they feel. This can either be calibrated with lines at centimetre points, or can be assessed during the analysis by laying over the line a clear piece of plastic that is calibrated. This approach is often used in relation to pain. An example would be:

Mark with a cross on the line how you would describe your pain now

Worst pain imaginable   No pain at all

The analysis of the responses

The analysis of both the Likert scale and the visual analogue scale can be treated in a similar way, by allocating a numeric value for the chosen response. In the case of the Likert scale a score of 5 can be allocated for 'strongly agree' answers, 4 for 'agree', 3 for 'neither agree/disagree', 2 for 'disagree' and 1 for 'strongly disagree' when the statement is in the positive. When the statement is expressed in the negative, the reverse order of numbering would be applied (i.e. strongly disagree to the statement 'the midwife did not have time to answer my questions' would be scored 5 to show there was a positive response to the midwife). An overall score for all the Likert questions can then be calculated for each person. It is also possible to give an average score for everyone in the sample. So for instance, an average of 4.2 for the statement *'I felt confident with the midwife who delivered me'* would suggest that there was a high degree of satisfaction as the average was between the 'agree' and 'strongly agree' point on the scale. In the same way the points on the visual analogue scale could be divided into ten sections with each section given a score from one to ten, where ten could be allocated to the positive end of the scale and one to the negative.

In questions requiring a 'yes' or 'no' answer, the responses can be expressed as a proportion of the total in terms of the percentage giving each response. The method of analysis should be carefully thought out at the design stage, and tested in the pilot and not left until the questionnaires start arriving.

Conducting research

Although a survey provides quick and easy access to a large amount of data, the researcher should be cautious in the use of the questionnaire. This is because it is not always appropriate for those for whom writing is either not an easy or welcome mental activity, or for those who have physical conditions, such as visual or writing problems. We also have to remember that even for those used to expressing themselves on paper, questionnaires have almost reached saturation point, and the motivation to complete and return a detailed questionnaire may be low.

Consideration must be given to the nature of the terms of reference, the sample under consideration, and the possible advantages of using an alternative method such as interviews. The question of ethics should also be raised at this stage, as thought needs to be given to the possible harm through upset, anxiety or guilt caused by certain kinds of topic areas. These may include the loss of a baby, or the birth of a baby with a medical problem that may be thought to relate to maternal behaviour, such as smoking or dietary intake. Robinson (1996) warns that personal questions can cause distress to patients and arouse anxieties that may linger. Care should be taken, then, where the respondent may confront emotionally sensitive issues when they may be in a vulnerable mental state, and may have no one to help them through the distress caused by the questionnaire.

Where the decision to use the questionnaire is appropriate, it is important to avoid believing it is all a matter of writing appropriate questions down on paper. The three elements of covering letter, instructions and main body of the questionnaire need careful planning and design. The review of the literature will help identify appropriate topic areas, and may even give some pointers as to the kind of questions that have worked well in other studies. In selecting the wording of the questions the researcher must keep validity and reliability in mind. The two important questions that need to be constantly addressed are:

- ◆ What am I trying to measure (validity)?
- ◆ How accurately will this question measure it (reliability)?

The basic principles of questionnaire design (Box 9.4) should then be rigorously followed. Decisions on how the data resulting from each question are to be presented in a report/article should be considered at the question design stage. If you feel you may need statistical advice, it is at this stage that it should be sought.

It is important to make the questions as clear and as straightforward as possible. This means using simple language and simple sentences. Midwifery or medical jargon and abbreviations should be avoided as much as possible. It is not easy for the researcher to spot vague terms and ambiguity as they have designed the question and are not confused on the meaning, so it is important to ask others to comment at the design stage.

A questionnaire should be interesting and enjoyable for your respondents to fill in. There should be variety in the way the questions are asked or require to be answered. The most frustrating experience for a respondent is to find that the choice of words clearly betrays the researcher's preconceived assumptions or personal agenda. This can be revealed through the use of emotive words such as 'better', 'disappointed', 'acceptable', and so on.

A pilot must be undertaken. In the pilot it is important to have a good cross-section of the kinds of people who will be included in the main study. This is perhaps just as important as the size of the sample. The main questionnaire should be accompanied with one asking pilot respondents to identify any particular strengths or weaknesses. Good questions include:

- How long did it take you to complete the questionnaire?
- Were there any questions you had particular problems with?
- Was there any particular wording you had difficulty with?
- Are there any questions you feel were missing from the questionnaire?
- To sum up; what did you feel were the strengths of the questionnaire?
- What areas do you feel could be presented differently?

It is a good idea to produce a report based on the analysis of the data from the pilot to provide experience of moving from raw data-to-data presentation and analysis. At this point serious shortcomings in the design of some questions, especially the method of answering, can be revealed.

This chapter has concentrated on the use of a written questionnaire; however, in the future more questionnaires will be sent using the Internet. New skills in designing suitable questionnaires will be required by researchers (Coombes 2001), but this medium may open up new possibilities in the collection of health data. Researchers must now pay more attention to the way in which computers can help with both the design and analysis of questionnaires. As technology advances, the use of Internet questionnaires will be a natural extension of this trend.

Critiquing research

Questionnaires are a popular method of data collection in midwifery. The danger is that we have become so familiar with them that we rarely stop and challenge their use. We do need to ensure that the researcher has given a clear rationale for the choice of questionnaire rather than the usually more effective method of interviewing. Where the sample is geographically spread, or where an existing relationship between the researcher and participants may compromise the use of interviews, then questionnaires are a good choice. It is worth thinking about any ethical issues raised by the use of the questionnaires, and whether the researcher has addressed these. For instance, we would be unhappy where a questionnaire was used to explore feelings about a still-birth or abortion, or similar subjects that may result in upset, anxiety or need-lessly raising feelings of guilt, confusion or regret.

The space provided in some journals does not permit the inclusion of an entire questionnaire, so we cannot always judge the quality of the design. Sometimes tables provide a clue as to the content and wording of the questionnaire. Where possible, place yourself in the position of the respond-ents and ask was there any possibility of ambiguity, or misunderstanding? Are the questions in any way leading, for instance, the use of emotive words that suggests how the researcher felt about the topic?

What evidence is there that the researcher addressed the issue of reliability of the questions, especially if they were designed for the study and had not been used in previous studies? Was the accuracy of the questions tested through a pilot study? In regard to validity, how do we know the questions were measuring what they were supposed to measure? Did the researcher develop some of the questions from previous research, or were experts in the field approached to comment on the appropriateness of the topics for the study?

Finally, we should consider the researcher's interpretation of the results. Are the results strong enough to support the statements made by the researcher? We should also be aware of the words/deeds dilemma, in that what people say they do, may not be what they do in practice. In other words we should always be somewhat cautious in treating self-report data as if it were 'the truth'.

Key Points

◆ Questionnaires enable a large amount of data to be collected quickly and cheaply. They have the advantage of being familiar to a majority of the population, and compared to other forms of data collection are a reasonably non-threatening medium for both the researcher and respondent.

◆ The response rate is variable. Where it falls under 50%, it is difficult to be certain that the responses received are representative of the sample that received it.

◆ Questionnaires have been used so much in the past that people are now less likely to return them. Serious consideration should be given as to whether this is the most appropriate method. In particular, the ethical issue of harm should be considered where the questions could produce emotional upset, regret, anxiety or confusion.

◆ Designing a questionnaire involves three elements: the covering letter, the instructions, and the body of the questionnaire. There are clear guidelines that should be followed in the construction of questions. The importance of avoiding bias and ensuring reliability and validity must be stressed.

◆ It should be remembered that the basic premise of questionnaire design is that the respondent can read and write, and is fluent in the English language. For one reason or another there is a proportion of the population who will always be excluded where questionnaires are used to collect research data.

◆ A pilot study is a good indicator of rigour in the use of questionnaires.

References

Burns N and Grove S (2001) The Practice of Nursing Research: Conduct, Critique, and Utilization (4th edn). Philadelphia: W.B. Saunders.

Coombes H (2001) Research Using IT. Houndmills: Palgrave.

Couchman W and Dawson J (1995) Nursing and Health-Care Research: A Practical Guide (2nd edn). London: Scutari.

Furber C (2000) An exploration of midwives' attitudes to health promotion. Midwifery 16(4): 314–322.

Holloway I and Fullbrook P (2001) Revisiting qualitative inquiry: Interviewing in nursing and midwifery research. NT Research 6(1): 539–50.

Lavender T, Moffat H and Rixon S (2000) Do we provide information to women in the best way? British Journal of Midwifery 8(12): 769–775.

LoBiondo-Wood G and Haber J (2002) Nursing Research: Methods, Critical Appraisal, and Utilization (5th edn). St Louis: Mosby.

Murphy-Black T (2000) Questionnaire. In: Cormack D (ed.) The Research Process in Nursing (4th edn). Oxford: Blackwell Science.

Polit D, Beck B and Hungler B (2001) Essentials of Nursing Research: Methods, Appraisal, and Utilization (5th edn). Philadelphia: Lippincott.

Robinson J (1996) 'It's only a questionnaire' ... ethics in social science research. British Journal of Midwifery 4(1): 41–44.

Singh D, Newburn M, Smith N and Wiggins M (2002) The information needs of first-time pregnant mothers. British Journal of Midwifery 10(1): 54–58.

Sarantakos S (1994) Social Research. Houndsmill: Macmillan.

CHAPTER TEN
Interviews

In the last chapter we ended by considering one of the two main methods of collecting survey data: the questionnaire. Although popular with researchers, this is not always the most appropriate choice for a number of reasons. One of their major problems is poor response rate associated with questionnaires. Certainly for the mothers of new babies, sitting down to complete a questionnaire may be difficult to achieve. Not only can questionnaires be difficult to fit into a hectic lifestyle, but also they are now almost an over-used medium for collecting research data. There is so much 'junk mail' received in the post that it is very easy to include questionnaires in this category.

The second main method of collecting data in surveys is the use of the interview. These have a great deal to offer midwifery research as the type of data it produces tends to be richer, and has more depth than is generally possible with questionnaires. Interviews also make use of the midwife's professional skill of sensitively collecting information through a conversational medium. It can also increase the range of people included in a study.

In this chapter we examine some of the features of interviews, especially their advantages and disadvantages, and pay particular attention to some of the skills involved in interviewing.

Definition

Interviews consist of data gathering through direct interaction between a researcher and respondent where answers to questions are gathered verbally. They can take the form of face-to-face encounters or the use of the telephone. Although usually conducted on a one-to-one basis, they can be carried out with a group of individuals in the form of focus groups. These are small groups of usually similar individuals who are prompted by the researcher to discuss certain topics and experiences. They have a certain degree of acceptability with participants, because, as McKie (1996) points out, they capitalize on the most natural form of social communication, the conversation.

Interview structure

Interviewing is a family of research approaches, according to Arksey and Knight (1999), that demand method more than common sense. In other words, the need to ensure validity and reliability means that attention must be paid to elements not normally associated with daily conversation and so require more thought than we might anticipate. One of the ways in which this family of approaches varies is in the degree of structure it contains. This can range from a highly structured format, where they virtually take the form of reading out questions from a questionnaire and recording the answers. This approach is used in survey designs that concentrate on the production of quantitative data (Newell 1994). Here, the list of questions is not called a questionnaire but an interview schedule. The advantages of this format are emphasized by Newell (1994) who suggests the following:

- It is easier to code the responses and analyze and interpret the data
- The uniformity of the questioning enables the results to be analyzed quantitatively and tested for statistical significance
- It is easier to train interviewers to use a structured interview schedule as written guidance on its use is provided
- Producing a structured interview schedule encourages the researcher to crystallize his or her thoughts and ensure that clear definitions and precise questions are developed.
  (p. 15)

The disadvantage of a highly structured approach is that there is little scope for spontaneity and depth of information. It can also be very superficial leaving us with little understanding of a situation. Newell (1994) also points out that of all interviewing techniques, the structured interview is the one that differs the most from normal conversational interaction. She also suggests that the disadvantages include omitting areas relevant to a study because the researcher has not considered them, and forcing respondents to choose from a list of closed options, none of which really apply.

At the other end of the interview continuum is the unstructured, or non-standardized interview, where the line of questioning develops very much as appropriate within a particular interview. The advantage of this approach is that the interviewer responds to the experiences or situation of the respondent, and the information is not forced or channelled into a limited number of options. In this way, as Arksey and Knight (1999) point out, the participants are encouraged to be open and spontaneous and to use their own words, expressions and ideas rather than those of the researcher. This means that whilst the participant is more active in terms of directing the flow of information, the researcher is more passive than is usual in interview situations. This form is particularly suited to situations where the researcher knows the broad area to be covered, such as the decision on the method of infant feeding, but is unsure of the exact points to be covered. Using a qualitative method, issues can be explored in an unrestricted manner and so illuminate the topic from the respondent's point of view (McKie 1996). This is a favoured design in qualitative research, as it allows the voice of the individual to be heard, and helps the researcher understand a phenomenon from the other person's perspective (Holloway and Fullbrook 2001).

The disadvantage of the approach is that this loose structure makes it very difficult to summarize a number of interviews together, as they may cover very different topics and issues. Analysis can thus be more difficult and time consuming.

In between these two extremes are semi-structured interviews that are a mixture of the two. They contain some standard questions that are asked of everyone, but there is also the flexibility to probe and explore areas that seem appropriate to the individual concerned. An interview guide is the name given to the checklist of questions, or key words used by the interviewer in this kind of situation. Coombes (2001) sees this approach as one of the best for the researcher because of this balance between structure to guide the overall interviews and the flexibility to react to the information and explore areas they may not have considered. This provides an opportunity to get closer to the accurate views, feelings and experiences of the participant and so enhance validity.

These three different forms of the interview are imaginary points along a continuum. Most interviews will not be located neatly at one of these points, but somewhere between the two extremes, depending on the nature of the research question and the way the researcher has decided to answer it.

Advantages of interviews

Why choose interviews as a data-collection method? There are a number of very clear advantages to using interviews as can be seen from Box 10.1. According to Polit et al (2001), the strengths of interviews far outweigh those of questionnaires. They have a higher response rate, are suitable for a wider variety of individuals than questionnaires, are less likely to lead to misinterpretations of the questions, and provide richer data than questionnaires. This is because the choice of answers usually has fewer restrictions than the visual prompts provided by questionnaires. The presence of the interviewer can also be an asset as they can encourage the provision of complete and accurate answers. This has been recognized by Burns and Grove (2001) who

---

- ◆ Participation can be gained from a wide range of people including those who have a problem with literacy, visual problems, and are suitable for mothers and health professionals who have little time to complete questionnaires
- ◆ Response rate is usually higher than questionnaires
- ◆ The interviewer can reduce misunderstandings and the number of missed questions
- ◆ Participants can feel more in control in semi-structured and unstructured interviews and therefore feel more valued
- ◆ Most of the data is usable
- ◆ In-depth responses can be gained
- ◆ Information is immediately available
- ◆ Overall better quality data in comparison to questionnaires.

Box 10.1 Advantages of interviews

◆ Interviewing is a highly skilled activity that requires careful training and practice
◆ It is time consuming and costly to carry out and analyze in comparison to questionnaires
◆ There is a danger of participants providing 'socially acceptable' answers
◆ Participants can be influenced by the interviewer's status, characteristics or behaviour
◆ Participants can feel put on the spot, 'tested', or worry they will 'look a fool' if they answer completely honestly
◆ Some participants may not be used to expressing their deep feelings or emotions openly to others.

Box 10.2 Disadvantages of interviews

suggest that interviews allow the researcher to explore a greater depth of meaning than can be obtained with other methods.

Interviews have a particular relevance in midwifery as they provide an opportunity to pursue a woman-centred approach to issues and situations. This is particularly the case in semi-structured and unstructured interviews as their purpose is to hear 'the voice' of the participants, so as to enable an understanding of the situation from their perspective (Holloway and Fulbrook 2001).

As with all the other methods of data collection presented in this book, we have to be aware of the disadvantages of interviews. The main issues are outlined in Box 10.2. A number of these relate to the practicalities of the technique. They require a great deal of time per interview in terms of both gathering the data and their analysis, particularly where the interview is semi-structured or unstructured.

The other main problem area is the influence of the interviewer. The fact that this is a social situation means that the characteristics of each of the individuals concerned can play a part in the reliability and validity of the information produced. There is inevitably a conscious or subconscious influence on the selection of information by the participant where the interviewer is a midwife, no matter how much they encourage participants to 'tell it as it is'. Hardy and Mulhall (1994) draw attention to this, and question the implication of interview situations where the interviewer is a health professional, and the participant a member of the public. They pose the question 'does the status of the interviewer influence the type of answer where the interviewer is seen as a powerful figure when socially desirable answers may be given?' Social desirability means that people say what they feel will show them in a positive light to the interviewer and people in general.

In the same way, a participant may provide a carefully thought out logical answer to a question rather than admit that they act on intuition, 'illogical' thinking or rely on serendipity in decision making. One final problem is where the participant 'second guesses' the answers on the basis of what they think the interviewer wants to hear. All these elements will have a negative effect on the validity of interview data.

Planning the interview

Interviewing is rather like marriage: everybody knows what it is, an awful lot of people do it, and yet behind each closed door is a world of secrets.

The above statement from the classic work on interviewing by Oakley (1981) illustrates why we need to examine the interview in detail. Interviewing is a skill frequently practised outside the gaze of those who need to learn from those who do it well. Although as a method of data collection asking questions and receiving answers sounds deceptively easy, like everything else in research, things are never that simple. It is possible, however, to overcome some of the difficulties through a knowledge of the pitfalls and follow a few basic principles.

A major step is to recognize that research interviews are not like ordinary conversations as their purpose is to elicit research data. Burns and Grove (2001) warn that nurses and midwives may feel that because they frequently use the interview in clinical assessments, the dynamics of the interview are familiar, however, they emphasize, using the technique for research requires greater sophistication. They go on to provide the following essential advice:

Developing skills in interviewing requires practice. Interviewers need to be very familiar with the content of the interview. They must anticipate situations that might occur during the interview and develop strategies for dealing with them.
(p. 421)

Their advice is for the interviewer to use role-play to develop appropriate skills and coping mechanisms. This should be firstly with colleagues, where it can be used very much like a rehearsal. These could be tape recorded or even videoed for playback later to identify appropriate skills and areas that need developing. This should, of course, be followed up later with a pilot study with members from the group in whom the researcher is interested.

A major consideration in carrying out an interview is the location and characteristics of the environment in which the interview takes place. The participant should feel relaxed and comfortable. There should be as few disturbances and distractions as possible whilst the interview takes place. Although many people provide the best information in their own home, the interviewer's control over the setting is drastically reduced. Despite interruptions having an impact on the flow of information, sometimes this has to be accepted and may be inevitable, especially with a young baby around. One student told me of a recent interview she had undertaken where there was not only a fierce-looking dog present, but also a rabbit running around. The woman being interviewed jumped up at one point to shoo away the rabbit that had urinated on the dog's bedding for the third time, while the dog sat in a corner vomiting. All of this was captured on audiotape. Under these circumstances it is important the interviewer does not show any irritation, exasperation, surprise or disgust.

Interviews in a participant's home does raise issues of personal safety, and it is wise for the researcher to take steps to ensure that people know where they are and the timetable they are following. The researcher should also protect themselves by carrying such items as a mobile phone and alarm, to enhance personal safety. Wherever the interview takes place, simple things such as ensuring that the sun is not shining in the participant's eyes, and that they are comfortable is important, as this will affect the quality of the information produced.

The interviewer's appearance also needs careful thought, if the possibility of producing socially desirable answers is to be minimized. The way the interviewer is dressed or the accessories they wear could act as distractions, or indications of possible personal beliefs and values. Where possible the interviewer's appearance should be relatively nondescript. In terms of etiquette, it is also important that the interviewer states the approximate length of time the interview may take and ensures that the respondent is not worried about other responsibilities or obligations that may distract them as the interview lengthens.

The nature of the interview will also be influenced by the method of recording the answers. The two options are making written notes as the interview unfolds, or using a tape recorder. Both have their advantages and disadvantages. Written notes are not as intimidating as using a tape recorder, and the interviewer is not worried by background noise. There is also little risk of technology letting the researcher down, although it is important to have a good supply of pens or pencils that are in good working order! The disadvantage of writing is the inability to maintain eye contact with participants. This can be a difficulty for both the interviewer and participant. It can feel somewhat like making a police statement rather than an interview. There is also an inevitable loss of information, as it is rarely possible to write down everything that is said. The main difficulty for the researcher is coping with a racing mind that is thinking of the next question, remembering what has just been said, trying to remember how to spell tricky words and making a mental note of interesting comments that have just been made that will need to be probed or followed up later.

Arksey and Knight (1999) point out that audiotaping is probably the most popular method of recording qualitative interviews. Tape recorders have the advantage of leaving the interviewer free to concentrate on the conversation rather than trying to speed-write everything that is said. The ability to maintain eye contact can also be very important in interviews on sensitive topics. Apart from the problem of background noise, tape recorders are successful in capturing almost all of the comments from the participant in their own words. This can be a crucial advantage, particularly in qualitative research. The disadvantages of tape recorders include the fact that some participants find them intimidating. They are an additional worry for the interviewer, in case something goes wrong with them, such as the tape jamming, or batteries running out. The resultant interviews can also take a long time to transcribe for analysis.

Interviewing skills

What makes a good interview? McKie (1996) suggests that there are a number of factors that can be divided into objective and subjective qualities of the interviewer. The objective qualities include the interviewer's age, gender, social class, manner of dress and accent. Subjective factors include the ability of the researcher to quickly establish rapport and maintain a smooth flow within the interview. Apart from choice of dress, there is little the interviewer can do about the objective qualities, so it is the subjective factors that require more detailed analysis.

Good interviews are the result of more than asking the questions clearly, although that does help. Arksey and Knight (1999), cite a newspaper report, revealing that 7% of the impact of any piece of communication is verbal, 37% comes from the tone of voice and 56% comes from body language. This emphasizes the complexity of the interview process. They suggest that being interested in others helps to sustain enthusiasm for the job of interviewing. Importantly, they also suggest that being self-aware makes a significant contribution to doing the job well. A number of additional ingredients of a skilled interview are provided by Coombes in the form of a checklist (see Box 10.3).

There are a number of elements that need to be mastered by the interviewer under the heading of non-verbal communication skills. Their purpose is to improve the establishment and maintenance of 'rapport', which can be defined as an understanding and close relationship between both parties. The physical position of the interviewer in relation to the participant is critical; if they are square-on, almost in a head-to-head position, the participant may feel it is more like an interrogation rather than a relaxed conversation. Sitting slightly to the side of the individual where eye contact can be made helps to establish the right atmosphere. It is important that this is at a comfortable distance from the individual, so that they do not feel that their personal space is being restricted or invaded.

Comfortable eye contact has already been identified as part of non-verbal skills and the researcher leaning slightly forward to indicate that they are listening enhances this. The interviewer should avoid crossing their arms or legs, which may suggest that they are nervous, or keeping certain information secret from the respondent. The key element is to relax. If the interviewer is relaxed, it will encourage the respondent to similarly relax.

- ◆ Strive to be non-judgemental
- ◆ Choose the right vocabulary
- ◆ Express an interest in what they are telling you
- ◆ Be aware of non-verbal communication
- ◆ Be silent when the participant pauses. They may need time to gather their thoughts
- ◆ Really listen to what they are telling you.

Box 10.3 Interview checklist (reproduced with permission from Coombes 2001 p. 103)

Closing the interview

◆ Leave people with a feeling of success, for instance indicate how valuable and insightful the observations generated have been
◆ Confirm what will happen next: how and when the results will be made available; whether participants will be offered the chance to check transcripts, or a draft of the research report; if and when people are likely to be contacted for follow-up work.

After the interview

◆ Write to thank the participant for taking part in the study.

Box 10.4   Closing the interview and afterwards (reproduced with permission from Arksey and Knight 1999 p. 102)

Two further elements relate to how the interviewer ends the interview and the contact they make with the participant following the interview. Suggestions relating to these have been made by Arksey and Knight (1999) and are presented in Box 10.4.

It is also important to add one more suggestion to the closing of the interview, and that is to offer the participant the opportunity to ask any questions of the interviewer. This allows any concerns or important questions to be identified, that may have come to the participant's mind during the course of the interview. These may be addressed by the researcher and may put their mind at ease. This is a clear demonstration of the kind of the reciprocity that should exist in interviews, where the researcher should share any expertise or knowledge with the participant.

When things go wrong

Inevitably things may go wrong during an interview, and it is just as well to be prepared for them. Common problems include an incomplete answer to a question, where the participant only gives part of an answer. Other problems include wrongly anticipating a question and so providing an answer that is not appropriate to the question. The following suggestions from a classic survey methods text by Moser and Kalton (1971) can be very useful techniques to correct the situation.

◆ Use of the expectant pause
◆ Use of the expectant glance
◆ Repeat part of the answer
◆ Repeat original question.
  (p. 277)

The first two suggestions of an expectant pause or glance suggest to the participant that it is still 'their turn' to speak, and this will usually be taken as a cue to continue with their conversation. However, care has to be taken, with both of these techniques, as the expectant pause can turn into an embarrassing silence, and the expectant glance can turn into a nervous twitch. Repeating part of the answer can also be a signal to continue, and is very useful when taking written notes, as it allows the participant to receive feedback that the information has been received by the researcher. Repeating the original question can alert the participant that perhaps the original question was misheard, and will allow them to correct this by providing an answer that corresponds with the question posed.

We should also remember that things could go wrong in an interview because it is potentially a stressful situation for both interviewer and participant. Both may suffer from what can be described as 'stage fright'. That is, they may restrict what they say or not act naturally because they are intimidated or overawed by their involvement in research. This feeling can be increased where a tape recorder is used. The participant's reaction to this situation can be quickly spotted when the interview becomes more like a quick question and answer session, rather than the establishment of a considered and in-depth answer. The replies may be very short one word or sentence answers, or the participant might keep saying they do not remember, or it never bothered them.

Some of the problem may lie with the interviewer. If intimidated they may hurry the interview along so the participant does not get sufficient time to reflect on the answer before the next question is asked. In this situation the interviewer needs practice in interviewing, so that they are comfortable with the technique. Where a tape recorder is used, it should be placed discreetly out of eye-line for both parties, so they are not intimidated by its presence.

All the issues in this section underline the conclusion that interviewing is a highly skilled activity. The interviewer should be familiar with the content of the interview, and should have practised with it several times before it is piloted under natural conditions. The rewards of interviews are many, and it is worth considering the way in which research based on interviews have illuminated many of the important issues in midwifery.

Conducting research

Interviews should be considered when the research question depends on a self-report that can be improved by a face-to-face situation. This can be where the individual may not have considered the subject in any depth or may not feel their views are important enough to return a questionnaire. Similarly, they should be considered where the topic might be one capable of great depth and a questionnaire would be too superficial a tool. They should also be considered where the researcher intends to explore the topic through the eyes of the participant and wants participants to recount their experiences in some depth in their own words. The more detail required in a study and the more depth required then the more likely it is that interviews are the tool of choice, either as the sole tool or as an addition to another tool such as observation.

Once the interview has been decided as the appropriate tool, the researcher must consider the degree of structure it will contain ranging from structured, through to semi-structured and unstructured. Whichever degree of structure, the researcher must ensure they are fully trained and experienced in undertaking the role of interviewer. Remember the advice above to rehearse with colleagues using a tape recorder, to listen to your strengths and areas that might need to be improved.

In the interview setting, it is important to be aware of the impact of interruptions and distractions. The body language of the interviewer is fundamental in helping the participant to relax in what can be a very stressful and intimidating situation. Although there are many skills involved in the interview, it is worth remembering the advice of Coombes (2001), to really listen and to avoid rephrasing the participant's answer in your own words, as this can lead to bias. Where it is clear that the participant has decided to follow one line of a description, or account, rather than another, it is imperative for the interviewer to consider whether they need to bring them back to that point and explore the other alternative. Where an interruption occurs the interviewer may have to help the respondent to return to the place that had been reached before the interruption.

Anything can happen in a free-flowing interview. An important word of warning is that while telling their 'story', respondents can relive painful memories, and experience heightened emotional responses. If a memory is stressful or painful, the respondent may exhibit anger, fear, sadness or upset. Under these circumstances the interview may have to be abandoned or delayed until the participant makes a decision as to whether they want to continue, or the interviewer feels that it would be in the participant's best interest to abandon or reschedule the session. However, some people find these emotional moments therapeutic. Participants can sometimes feel grateful for the opportunity for someone at last to listen to and acknowledge their experiences and feelings.

Where an interview is particularly intense, it is possible for the feelings of closeness with the interviewer to lead to the participant revealing 'secret information'. It should be remembered that where the interviewer is a midwife, the professional code of conduct does not allow all information to be kept secret. Examples would be anything related to a child or mother, abuse or neglect, or a report of poor professional conduct. Under these circumstances the midwife cannot adopt a researcher role of keeping the information confidential but has a duty to report it. If the situation arises where a participant indicates that they want to share something that they indicate is particularly confidential, the midwife interviewer must stop them and make their own position clear before the participant says something that they may later regret (see Chapter 8 on ethics).

These points emphasize the exhausting nature of interviews, especially those touching on very sensitive areas. It is possible for the researcher to absorb a great deal of other people's emotional baggage that must then be dealt with. For this reason it is important to avoid conducting more than a small number of interviews a day and to have a good research supervisor or mentor who can help deal with the emotional after-effects of interviewing in a positive way.

Finally, at the end of the interview Morse and Field (1996) suggest that the interview should end with the questions 'Is there anything you would like to ask me?' and 'Is there anything else I should have asked you?'

Critiquing research

In critiquing a research article that has used interviews, the first question to ask is, 'was it an appropriate choice of data-collection tool?' In other words, would the disadvantages of the interview have suggested that an alternative method might have been more appropriate?

One problem with many research reports is that it is difficult to get an idea of the conditions under which the interview took place. We frequently have no idea of the possible strength and weakness that may have influenced the reliability of the interview. An excellent exception is the work of Bluff and Holloway (1994) where a great deal of detail is provided on the environment in which the interviews took place, and the details of the interviews themselves. Studies published more recently do not have the same amount of rich detail on the interviewing process as this work.

In most instances, although the person undertaking the interview may be named, we have little idea of their appearance at the time of the interviews, and how they were dressed. If the interviewer was a midwife, did the participants know them, and were they in uniform? Both these factors may influence the results.

We also need some indication of the degree of structure in the interview that may have encouraged or curtailed the views of the respondent, and the language in which they could respond; the more the interview was structured, the less it is possible to express views in the participant's own words.

The presentation of results is also important. Although some selection and editing is inevitable, the more that has taken place, the less authentic the results. Even with some editing, however, it is possible to retain the feelings and emotions of the participants, as the following extract from Ng and Sinclair (2002) demonstrates. The dotted lines indicate where some words have been edited out and the square brackets '[' indicate where the author has added some words of clarification.

> *Of the births, no two were anyway the same ... It was great, I remember seeing the baby when she was born ... and thinking Oh, she's so beautiful [first home birth] ... The feeling when he was born was just sheer relief (laughs) [second home birth] ... then when it came to the next baby, that's when I had "the" home birth experience that people talked about (laughs), it was very different ... it was a gorgeous ... birth, I thoroughly enjoyed it [third home birth] ... Anyway, the birth wasn't a picnic again [fourth home birth] ... The last one was very messy [fifth home birth].*
> (p. 58)

There is no doubt that we can 'hear' the voice of the woman speaking here, and the emotions she was conveying about her home deliveries. This would not have been the same had it been the result of ticked boxes on a questionnaire.

An important note on which to end is the reminder that interviews and questionnaires only relate to what people say, and not necessarily to what they do. The relationship between words and actions remains problematic. We would need further evidence in the form of observational data to convince us that people do what they say they do.

Key Points

♦ As a means of data collection, interviews have many advantages over questionnaires. In midwifery they also have the advantage that they are compatible with a woman-centred approach to care. They can be used to collect quantitative data using a structured interview schedule, or qualitative data using a semi-structured, or unstructured format.

♦ Semi-structured, and unstructured interviews have the advantage that they can collect a rich quantity of data through the prolonged and interactive format of the interview. They provide a unique view of events as seen by those receiving services, or those experiencing parenthood. The results are frequently unexpected, illuminating, and can differ from the perspective of health professionals.

♦ There are a number of disadvantages to interviews. They are costly and time consuming. The physical presence of the researcher can also be intimidating to some participants, and the resulting data can be consciously or subconsciously skewed in the direction of socially desirable answers. They also require a high level of skill on the part of the interviewer to avoid some of the pitfalls outlined.

♦ The time-consuming nature of interviews means that sample size is frequently smaller than that possible with questionnaires. However, this does not necessarily automatically limit their usefulness, especially where we are talking about qualitative research.

References

Arksey H and Knight P (1999) Interviewing for Social Scientists: An Introductory Resource with Examples. London: Sage.

Bluff R and Holloway I (1994) 'They know best': women's perception of midwifery care during labour and childbirth. Midwifery 10(3): 157–164.

Burns N and Grove S (2001) The Practice of Nursing Research: Conduct, Critique, and Utilization (4th edn). Philadelphia: W.B. Saunders.

Coombes H (2001) Research Using IT. Houndmills: Palgrave.

Hardy M and Mulhall A (1994) Nursing Research: Theory and Practice. London: Chapman and Hall.

Holloway I and Fullbrook P (2001) Revisiting qualitative inquiry: Interviewing in nursing and midwifery research. NT Research 6(1): 539–50.

McKie L (1996) Researching Women's Health: Methods and Process. Snow Hill: Quay books.

Morse J and Field P (1996) Nursing Research: The Application of Qualitative Approaches (2nd edn). London: Chapman and Hall.

Moser C and Kalton G (1971) Survey Methods in Social Investigations (2nd edn). London: Heinemann.

Newell R (1994). The structured interview. Nurse Researcher 1(3): 14–22.

Ng M and Sinclair M (2002) Women's experience of planned home birth: a phenomenological study. RCM Midwives Journal 5(2): 56–59.

Oakley A (1981). Interviewing women: a contradiction in terms. In: Roberts H (ed.) Doing Feminist Research. London: Routledge and Kegan Paul.

Polit D, Beck B and Hungler B (2001) Essentials of Nursing Research: Methods, Appraisal, and Utilization (5th edn). Philadelphia: Lippincott.

CHAPTER ELEVEN

Observation

In the last two chapters questionnaires and interviews have been described as methods that try to establish what people do and think by asking them directly. One of the major shortcomings of these two methods is that we have to assume that what people say they do is what they do in practice. Observation differs in that it collects information first hand based on what people are seen to do by the researcher.

The aim of this chapter is to consider the reasons for using observation as a method, and to identify some of its advantages and disadvantages. Two approaches to observation will be highlighted. Firstly, checklist observation will be briefly mentioned and then secondly, qualitative approaches to observation will be outlined in more detail. Although observation is used less frequently than questionnaires and interviews, there are a number of classic observational studies in midwifery, and some of these will be mentioned later. One of the main purposes of the chapter is to demonstrate that there is more to observation than meets the eye!

What is observation?

We are observing the world around us all the time, so how can we distinguish from a research perspective the difference between 'looking' and 'observing'? The answer according to LoBiondo-Wood and Haber (2002) is that observation in research is characterized by an emphasis on the objective and systematic nature of the process. They suggest that the researcher is not merely looking at what is happening, but rather is watching with a trained eye for certain specific events. They propose that observation should fulfil the following conditions:

1. The observations undertaken are consistent with the study's specific objectives.
2. There is a standardized and systematic plan for the observation and the recording of data.
3. All of the observations are checked and controlled.
4. The observations are related to scientific concepts and theories.
   (p. 298)

This list supports the view of Burns and Grove (2001) that observation is not a simple activity, no matter how easy we might think it is to 'look'. In a research context it is a method of describing events and situations in the real world. Observation can be defined as the collection of data that are visible to visual sensors, whether that consists of the researcher's eyes or the use of video.

As with interviews, the nature of the observation can vary depending on the amount of structure used to record the data. At one extreme is the highly structured observation checklist that leads to quantitative data, and at the other is the less-structured narrative description of events used to produce qualitative data.

Why use observation?

Although we can ask people what they do, we may not always get an accurate answer. This is because people are not always aware of what they do or are unable to accurately describe their actions. Some actions are carried out at a subconscious level and are difficult to explain verbally or write down. Explaining how to tie a shoelace over the phone is an example of this. This leads LoBiondo-Wood and Haber (2002) to conclude that observation is particularly suitable in complex research situations that are best viewed as total entities, and that are difficult to measure in parts. This applies to numerous midwifery activities where the best way to find out how someone does something is to watch them do it.

In conclusion, Polit et al (2001) state the argument for the use of observation as follows:

> ...virtually no other data collection method can provide the depth and variety of information as observation. With this approach, humans–the observers–are used as measuring instruments and provide a uniquely sensitive and intelligent (if fallible) tool.
> (p. 286)

Checklist observation

In checklist observation the researcher itemizes the kinds of activities to be observed, and then places a tick alongside that element each time it is occurs, for example, a checklist of the times in an antenatal class a midwife asks those present a direct question as a way of gaining involvement. The results are usually presented numerically, in the form of quantitative data.

Burns and Grove (2001) warn that care needs to be taken when drawing up the list of behaviours or activities to make sure that the categories do not overlap. An additional problem is where the observer must make a large number of inferences regarding a category such as 'gives emotional support'. The greater the degree of inference required, they suggest, the more difficult the category system is to use. The desired behaviours for checklist observation then, must be explicitly defined so that there is no question in the mind of the observer as to whether or not they occur. In other words clear concept definitions must be developed at the start of the study to ensure the accuracy of the recording.

As events and activities unfold so quickly, there is a limit to the number of different aspects the researcher can observe at once. Care has to be taken to avoid the checklist becoming too complex. For example, it may not be possible to accurately record the type, duration and form of touch between a midwife and woman in labour, as well as the duration of eye contact, and non-verbal forms of interaction.

Not only should the number of elements be considered in the checklist, but also the form of recording must be simplified to enable speed and accuracy. Simple ticks or crosses are the best form of recording items. Before using a checklist the researcher should thoroughly practise with a pilot study. This may suggest ways of reducing the complexity of the list, as well as providing the researcher with an opportunity to develop the skill of observing and recording at the same time.

The limitation of an observational checklist is the depth of information that can be achieved, and the limited complexity of interactions that can be accurately observed. This type of approach is also restricted to predicted behaviour, and does not cope well with unexpected activities not included on the checklist. This means it is easy to miss certain forms of behaviour because they have not been anticipated (Brink and Wood 1994).

Participant and non-participant observation

Anthropologists and sociologists first developed qualitative observational approaches to examine the actions and interactions of people in their natural social world. The classic typology of roles an observer may adopt when carrying out data collection was developed by Gold (1958) cited in Holloway and Wheeler (1996). This can be seen in Box 11. 1. The different roles vary in the extent to which the researcher becomes directly involved with those observed, that is whether the role is participant or non-participant. A further variation is

---

◆ **Complete participant.** The researcher is part of the setting and carries out covert observation as an 'insider'
◆ **Participant as observer.** Observation is overt and is carried out by the researcher who is an insider or has negotiated access to work alongside those in the setting and observe
◆ **Observer as participant.** In this situation the researcher is in the setting but does not have any real involvement with the activities that take place there, the emphasis is on the observation, which is overt
◆ **Complete observer.** Here the researcher is at a distance from the setting and what goes on there, and is unnoticed by those who are the subject of the research. Although this can take place unobtrusively from a close vantage point in the setting, such as in a reception area, it is usually applied to a two-way mirror situation, or video link.

Box 11.1 Gold's typology of observer role (reproduced with permission from Holloway and Wheeler, 1996:62)

the extent to which the observed are aware that they are being watched. The term *'overt'* signifies that those in the setting are aware of the observer's role, and *'covert'* to situations where they do not know that observation is taking place. LoBiondo-Wood and Haber (2002) use the term concealment and no concealment to describe these two situations. The more unstructured approach to observation consists of the researcher collecting data either as a participant or non-participant observer, or some variation in between.

There are few examples of the complete participant role being adopted in midwifery. An illustration provided by Phillips (1996) would be a midwife who joins an early pregnancy class as a client with the intentions of observing what goes on, and does not reveal she is both a midwife and researcher. Phillips rightly raises the ethical problems of this kind of deception, although it can be seen that once the identity and purpose of the observer is known, the accuracy of the data obtained may be affected as those involved know that everything is being recorded.

Perhaps one of the most frequently used roles is that of observer as participant. Here, interaction takes place with those who are being observed, and the role of researcher is clearly visible and agreed. One example is provided by Richens (2002) who carried out her ethnographic research 'to understand midwifery and client culture through the direct examination of behaviour and perceptions within a clinical setting'. As with many studies using observation, a variety of tools was used. Hers included participant and non-participant observation, tape-recorded interviews and clinical and patient records. The fieldwork data were collected over a six-month period in a British maternity unit. The role of observation and its advantage can be seen from the following extract:

> *Observation was the starting point for noting the behaviour of midwives. This allowed the author to see what was happening in practice and avoid biases inherent in participants' reports.*
> (p. 12)

One of the classic studies of ethnographic research in midwifery was carried out by Davies (1996). Her work provides a fund of detail about the process of observation and the role and experiences of the researcher in conducting observational research. The aim of her study was:

> *... to examine the differences and similarities between nursing and midwifery through the eyes of a set of student midwives, and to understand ways in which they attempted to 'make sense' of their new world.*
> (p. 88)

In this study, the role of the researcher as observer is made clear to the students who gave their permission to be observed. The study involved Davies in attending lectures and informal activities such as coffee and lunch breaks. The intention of such a study is not to see such activities as a researcher, but to see them through the eyes of those in the setting.

A further classic example of an ethnographic study is that of Hunt and Symonds (1995), where Hunt explored the culture of two maternity units over a six-month period. The aim of the study was to understand the culture, work practices and strategies of midwives. As with most ethnographic studies the interpretation of the role of observer was not static. Hunt appears to take on the role at times of participant as observer. This can be seen in the following passage.

> *The maternity unit was frequently very busy and the staff seemed happy to cast me in the role of someone who was an additional pair of hands with some inquisitive and quirky habits (note-taking, etc.) ... I was on the outside and on the inside at the same time, and never really 'at home'. The role is somewhere between stranger and friend.*
> (p. 46)

Both these classic studies have much in common, and illustrate the richness of data developed through ethnographic work. They contrast clearly with checklist observational studies in that the researcher is interested in more in-depth information that does not necessarily follow a clearly anticipated path. There is also a great emphasis on discovering the form of behaviour found in natural settings, such as a labour ward, or school of midwifery studies.

Perhaps in no other form of data collection does the researcher have to consider so carefully their role as researcher, as they play a total and often very visible role within the setting. This is illustrated by Hunt (Hunt and Symonds 1995) who at one point has to consider the consequence of answering the ward phone when it rings. She initially decides not to, as this may involve her too much in changing what would have taken place if she had not been there. There is also the danger that performing one activity will adversely affect the role of observer, so for instance she comments:

> *I did not feel I was capable of being a full-time ethnographer and full-time telephonist.*
> (p. 51)

Both Hunt and Davies plan carefully the clothes they will wear as researchers. Hunt decides in the early stages to wear a white coat, and comments that:

> *For someone in a white coat it appeared that access was unrestricted.*
> (p. 45)

Later this is abandoned once people in the setting are used to her presence, as she felt there was an element of deception in being mistaken for someone 'medical'.

Davies (1996) illustrates the same degree of thought in relation to what she wears in the company of the midwifery students. She describes her decision as follows:

> *I had been careful to choose something relatively unobtrusive from my wardrobe of formal and informal clothing. A simple blouse and skirt and warm sweater seemed to me to be most appropriate for 'fitting in' with the students*

*and not the 'uniform' associated with the 'establishment' (I normally wore a
smart suit and blouse when visiting as a professional officer).*
(p. 92)

The style of dress can have a profound effect on the way people may react in
a situation to someone as researcher. These are not, therefore, trivial details,
but are important elements the researcher has included in an attempt to
demonstrate credibility, where there is an attempt to share with the reader
the nature of the researcher's presence in the research environment.

Recording in observational studies

This section will concentrate on recording in qualitative observational
studies. Checklist designs are easier to imagine, as they consist of columns
in which a tick is placed if an activity or event is observed. Qualitative
observational methods are more complex, and raise more issues for the
researcher.

It is tempting to think of observation as simply watching what is happening and only using the sense of sight as the method of collection data. This is
far from accurate. Streubert and Carpenter (1999) point out that observation
is not intended to mean merely 'looking at' on the part of the researcher.
They stress that observation entails looking, listening, asking questions and
collecting artifacts. This last term means including objects that people make
or use. In ethnographic studies it frequently takes the form of diaries that
subjects may be asked to keep, as in the case of Davies (1996) where she
asked the students to keep a diary of their thoughts and experiences.

Fieldnotes are the major form of recording observations in qualitative
studies. These are narrative accounts of events and situations and can be
made while activities are in progress, or they can be written up some time
later. Each alternative has its advantages. The researcher may draw attention
to themselves if they write their observations during events, however, there
is a greater dependency on the accuracy of memory where notes are written
up later.

Davies (1996) reveals her strategy for recording fieldnotes, along with
some of the problems she encountered as follows:

*I kept detailed field notes, which was relatively easy to accomplish in an unob-
trusive fashion during classroom activities, but less so during the coffee and
lunch breaks and clinical sessions. I recorded the unsolicited interviews as
soon after the event as possible. Sometimes I even made notes quickly in the
toilet until I discovered Sian and Denise often waited for me, chatting at the
washbasins before leaving.*
(p. 95)

A similar strategy is used by Hunt (Hunt and Symonds 1995) and illustrates
the amount of data generated in ethnographic studies. Again in the following description the aim is to allow the reader to feel as though they
are in the setting and can follow the way in which the data are generated.

Hunt describes her recording activities as follows:

> *My data collection took a variety of forms. The main activity was the produc-*
> *tion of field notes. During the visit I would use my notebook to record head-*
> *ings and key phrases that would help me in the recording. I also used the*
> *dictaphone, usually in the toilet or store cupboard, to record key phrases and*
> *prompts. After each visit, when I returned home, I would write detailed field*
> *notes on the events of that visit. These were initially filed in date order. The*
> *field notes would include details of events and accounts of conversations.*
> *Much of the time was spent observing and informal interviewing those who*
> *had emerged as key informants. These interviews were unstructured and*
> *in the early days I recorded as much as possible of what was said, how it was*
> *said, to whom and on what occasions. The field notes also include lengthy*
> *descriptions of the labour ward, the office, the admission room, etc.*
> (p. 47)

These two descriptions provide a comprehensive account of how recording is achieved in a qualitative observational study. Unfortunately, the few recently published studies using observation do not contain this wealth of information.

Advantages

Observation is the most appropriate way of collecting research data in many situations, as the researcher is able to see what actually happens, and does not depend on reports that may be distorted by memory or perception. In checklist studies the frequency of events can be quantified, and relationships and correlation can be established.

It is in the area of qualitative research that observation can be particularly appropriate to midwifery research. This is especially true where an attempt is made to see things from the point of view of those receiving care. Morse and Field (1996) suggest that observation adds breadth to research and provides answers to contextual questions that cannot be answered by interview alone. The important point is that as observation takes place in a natural setting, it can provide an accurate picture of what actually happens. It can also take into account quite a large canvas of activity in the form of a description of, for example, a delivery spread over a long time period. Qualitative observation also provides flexibility, in that the focus of attention can change as a result of early observations.

The works of Kirkham (1989) and Hunt (Hunt and Symonds, 1995) are two classic examples of observational studies where the environment of midwifery activities is clearly described in a way that has a familiar realism attached to it. Each, however, provide insights that may go unnoticed by those used to working in those particular areas, as they have become 'unremarkable' occurrences.

Observational studies are not frequently found in midwifery, although they clearly have a lot to offer in gaining answers to questions that are not amenable to other forms of data collection. As with interviews, they can be used in both a quantitative and qualitative approach, and appear to be eminently suitable for midwifery research either as a single method or in conjunction with other forms of data collection.

Problems in observation

Despite the positive aspects of this method, there are a number of pitfalls. Ethical problems are a major concern for the qualitative researcher, especially where covert observation is being used. The issue is one of observing individuals who have not given their permission to be included in a study. This goes against the basic principles of informed consent discussed in Chapter 8.

However, one of the difficulties in observation is the problem of reactivity when people who are told what is being observed may change their normal behaviour. Take, for instance, the example given in Chapter 8 of observing student midwives hand-washing techniques and imagine indicating to a student that their technique is about to be observed. The result may be that their technique is surprisingly good! The observer is likely to be involved in very lengthy observations but probably these would be far from an accurate picture of normal activity.

Although LoBiondo-Wood and Haber (2002) agree that observing subjects without their knowledge violates the principle of informed consent, they suggest that sometimes there is no other way to collect such data, and where the data collected are unlikely to have negative consequences for the subject, the disadvantages of the study may be outweighed by the advantages. They suggest that *debriefing* is a possible way out of this dilemma by revealing the nature of the study after the observation and providing the opportunity for individuals to withhold their data from the study, and to discuss any questions they may have about the study.

A more acceptable answer may be to avoid open deceit by saying, in the case of the student midwife, that routine practices are to be observed, and for data collection to include other activities rather than simply hand washing.

The question of ethics is also raised in situations where the observer sees an activity that may put individuals at risk, or is an unprofessional act carried out by a member of staff. Although the researcher tries to maintain a confidential relationship with subjects, in certain circumstances it is not possible to honour this. One example would be where the observer has a public duty to disclose information as in the case of observing something unlawful or that may potentially put a child at risk. A second example would be where an observed activity relates to a breach of the code of professional practice, for example where the activity of another midwife was judged unsafe or putting health at risk (UKCC 1998). In both these examples the researcher is obliged to report these situations, and must abandon the researcher hat for that of the midwife (see Chapter 8 for a discussion of these issues).

From a practical point of view, observation is a very time consuming, and therefore expensive method. It also requires a great deal of interpersonal skills on the part of the observer, who should have training and experience with this method. Where more than one person is involved with the data gathering, there is also the problem of inter-observer reliability. This concerns the extent to which different observers select, interpret and record events in different ways.

One of the most obvious problems already referred to is that of *reactivity* (Polit et al 2001), that is, the extent to which the observer influences the activities of those observed. Kirkham (1989) draws attention to this in her work that looked at information giving between midwives and labouring women:

> *Inevitably, my presence affected what I observed. With midwives this initially had the effect of putting them on their best behaviour. I was quite happy with this as I wanted to know what behaviour these midwives saw as 'best' I discounted the observations of my first few hours where conversation was full of effusive 'pleases', 'thank you's and 'excuse me's'.*
> (p. 119)

This seems an inevitable feature of observations made in the early stages of a study, or in early interactions with individuals. A similar situation is recorded by Hunt (Hunt and Symonds 1995):

> *During the early fieldwork stages (the first two or three weeks) it was clear that the staff were making a very special effort to be good communicators. One midwife asked if I would tape her as she encouraged or coached a woman in the second stage of labour. It was an outstanding, energetic performance, worthy of its tape-recording and the language will be familiar to many midwives... The performance seemed to call for an applause, and the midwife smiled and seemed almost to bow at the end. She asked if that was what my research was all about. She explained she thought she was a good communicator and I should put this in my research. I promised I would.*
> (p. 46)

Both these extracts demonstrate the issue of validity. The observer has to consider the extent to which the observations are a true picture of what is going on. The 'ironic' tone of both authors' descriptions indicate that it is usually clear to the researcher when observations are not a true reflection of activities.

This challenge to both the reliability of the method, and validity of the results is reduced where the observation is spread over a longer time period where people relax more into their usual way of behaving.

Phillips (1996), drawing on the work of Gans (1982), points out that a further problem is the way the researcher will tend to like certain people in the study, and feel less comfortable with others. This can result in a 'gravitation' towards certain people and an avoidance of others that may influence the recording process. The best that the researcher can do is to be aware of this through their analysis of the fieldnotes, and attempt to redress the balance. The opposite of this is also true; some people in an observational study will like the researcher, and be willing to spend time with them, and be 'honest' with them. Others, for whatever reason, will feel less positive towards the researcher and will be less a source of accurate observational and interview material. This situation is not easy to sort out, as frequently the researcher is unaware of it.

Polit et al (2001) identify a number of concerns regarding the barriers to the researcher achieving objectivity in the conduct and analysis of field data. These include the following:

◆ Emotions, prejudices, and values of the observer may result in faulty inference.

◆ Personal interest and commitment may colour what is seen in the direction of what the observer wants to see.

◆ Anticipation of what is to be observed may affect what is observed.

◆ Hasty decisions before adequate information is collected may result in erroneous classifications or conclusion.
(p. 286)

A further problem for the midwife researcher is the difficulty of being able to stand back from the familiar taken-for-granted routine of the maternity setting, and ask 'why do things happen like this?' In anthropological terms, this is called establishing *'cultural strangeness'* where the aim is to see things from an outsider's point of view.

The longer the researcher is in the field, however, the greater the danger of what is referred to as *'going native'*. This term also comes from anthropological studies where, over an extended period of observing tribes, the researcher would become so at home with the new culture that they stop seeing activities and customs as 'strange' or noteworthy. In qualitative research, it refers to the researcher becoming over-familiar with the research setting and no longer noticing the kind of elements that need to be included in the observations (Morse and Field 1996).

A major problem for the researcher is one of selectivity. It is not possible to observe everything that is going on, or see things from every angle, decisions have to be made on where the observer will place themselves, and what they will attempt to observe. This will inevitably lead to some things being observed and others left out. In the same way, it is not possible to record everything, and some details will be omitted (Brink and Wood 1994).

In some situations there is also the possibility of misinterpreting what is going on. This is particularly true when observing a long established relationship where subtle patterns of communication styles have been developed and understood between people. These can appear strange or alien to the observer. The difference between cajoling someone to do something and apparently being hostile or unsympathetic can be easily misinterpreted by the researcher unaware of the usual pattern of conversation between people.

Observer bias is a further concern, where the researcher may be inclined to look out for certain activities and ignore others that do not fit in with their views or expectations. Where each period of observation is lengthy, *observer drift* can also be a problem, where the observer loses concentration, and finds themselves thinking of other things, and losing awareness of what is happening. In some situations, time sampling is carried out so that the day is broken down into shorter segments, and the researcher attempts to sample across all the time periods. This allows the researcher to remain relatively fresh throughout the period of observation. Where the researcher is concentrating on events, such as a delivery, this is not always a viable alternative, and an awareness of the danger of observer drift is the only precaution possible.

This range of possible pitfalls illustrates the complexity of this method. A number of excellent examples of qualitative research using observation exist in midwifery, all of which help the novice researcher to be aware of the problems.

Conducting research

As with each of the methods of research covered so far, the researcher must ensure that observation is the appropriate choice for the study terms of reference. In situations where self-reports may be inaccurate, or where there is a need to consider a total process or situation, then observation may be the best method to employ.

The decision on which type of observation should be selected is based on the nature of the research question. Where the question relates to a quantification of results, such as 'how often' or 'how much', or where the question is related to establishing whether something happens or not and with what frequency, a checklist design will be called for. This will take the form of a structured sheet that looks like a spreadsheet or grid, to allow ease of completion in the form of ticks, code numbers, or letters.

Where the research question does not imply a quantitative approach, but is more concerned with developing a broad understanding of how people act in a natural setting, as in an ethnographic study, then a participant, or non-participant observation study should be designed.

The exact role the researcher will play in this kind of research will require a great deal of thought. The variation in role from participant to non-participant observer should be considered (see Box 11.1). This does not necessarily mean that the researcher will stick to the one role. As Streubert and Carpenter (1999) comment, explicit rules for when to participate and when to observe are not available. The consequences of the different types of researcher role, however, must be considered in relation to their influence on those observed and the effect that this will have on the data gathered.

At an early point the ethical implications of the study need to be considered. Where an ethics committee (REC) is involved, informed consent, and the issue of possible deception should be addressed in a way that will satisfy the committee that consent has been considered, and harm will be avoided.

There are a large number of skills required of the observer. Phillips (1996), for instance, suggests that the observer needs to have good communication skills and a finely tuned sense of 'balance' to maintain what she refers to as 'that marginal yet crucial position of being at one and the same time both participant and observer'.

Hunt (Hunt and Symonds 1995) elaborates on the skills required of the ethnographer by saying:

Ethnography makes use of basic skills such as listening, watching, asking questions and the skills of 'sussing out'.
(p. 40)

By this she means that the researcher has to try and work out what is going on in a situation without using their own stereotypes and preconceptions. Rather, they should try and see things through the eyes of those observed. In terms of the practical activities concerned, DePoy and Gitlin (1994) list three essential activities of i) watching, ii) listening and iii) recording.

This last point raises the issue of what to record, and how. It is important in observation to have clear concept definitions for the items that will be recorded. This is true of checklist observation, as well as qualitative observational approaches. Polit et al (2001) provide a useful checklist of questions that can be used by the observer in planning which items need to be considered for inclusion in the study (see Box 11.2).

The form of recording will depend on the extent to which contemporary recording may disrupt the flow of activities being observed. The main alternatives will be note taking at the time or some time later, or the use of a dictaphone or tape recorder. DePoy and Gitlin (1994) make the following useful suggestion regarding how the observer should go about recording

---

1. **The physical setting – 'where' questions.** Where is the activity happening? What are the main features of the physical setting? What is the context within which human behaviour unfolds?
2. ***The participants – 'who' questions.*** Who is present? What are the characteristics of those present? How many people are there? What are their roles? Who is given free access to the setting – who 'belongs'? What brings these people together?
3. ***Activities – 'what' questions.*** What is going on? What are the participants doing? Is there a discernable progression of activities? How do the participants interact with one another? What methods do they use to communicate, and how frequently do they do so?
4. ***Frequency and duration – 'when' questions.*** When did the activity begin and end? Is the activity a recurring one and, if so, how regularly does it recur? How typical of such activities is the one under observation?
5. ***Process – 'how' questions.*** How is the activity organized? How are people interacting and communicating? How does the event unfold?
6. ***Outcomes – 'why' questions.*** Why is the activity happening, or why is it happening in this manner? What kinds of things will ensue? What did not happen (especially if it ought to have happened) and why?

Box 11.2   What to observe (reproduced with permission from Polit et al 2001:282)

fieldnotes:

> It is often helpful to think of yourself as a video camera and to record what the video camera would see as it scans the boundaries of the research. This technique reminds the researcher that description, not interpretation, is the first step in participant observation.
> (p. 220)

The exact details of what is recorded will change during the course of observation. Early notes may he very broad, and will try to establish some ideas of the kind of pattern of activity taking place. They will then become more focused depending on earlier observations, and the questions arising from the fieldnotes. Hunt (Hunt and Symonds 1995) provides an insight into the content of early fieldnotes as follows:

> The field notes were generally descriptive accounts of events observed in the field. Direct quotations were included whenever possible as were descriptions of such aspects as the tone of voice and the body language of the contributor. The field notes also included sketches of some aspects of the environment and maps to remind me of the layout of the unit.
> (p. 48)

The analysis stage of this kind of data is a very sophisticated activity. As with the analysis of quantitative data, advice and help should be sought from those with experience of this type of data.

In presenting the qualitative report or article, the structure is very different from that of a quantitative report or article. Some of the sources of work referred to in this chapter should be considered as a guide for writing the report in order to do full justice to the information collected.

Critiquing research

In critiquing observational research articles, we have to decide whether this was a suitable method to answer the research question. It is important to determine what the researcher was observing and how. In both checklist and qualitative approaches, does the researcher give a clear concept definition for the items being observed?

Did an ethics committee approve the study? Was the research overt or covert, that is, were people aware that they were being observed or not? Was permission sought from subjects where it was overt? Where permission was not sought, does the researcher provide a convincing justification for not securing this?

Where the researcher is active in the research setting, we must consider the extent to which they may have had an influence on the people and events observed. What did the researcher do to try to minimize the reactive effect on subjects? In good qualitative studies we should expect the researcher to provide a clear description of how they presented themselves in the setting in terms of dress and behaviour.

The role the researcher decided to play is important in deciding the extent to which people in the setting may have reacted to them. Which of the possible roles did the researcher select, and does this appear to have been a good choice? Did the researcher appear to display any bias, emotions, and prejudices in their dealings with those observed which may have influenced the quality of the data collected? Does the researcher appear to gravitate towards certain people in the study, and avoid others? In other words has there been a bias in who was observed that might have produced untypical results?

Where more than one observer was responsible for the data collection, how was inter-observer reliability achieved? Even where there is only one observer, it is important to establish if any training was received or a pilot study undertaken. An excellent example is set by Davies (1996) who took her research supervisor to her pilot study of a group of students attending a study day. She then compared her fieldnotes with those of the experienced supervisor.

Has the researcher included other methods of data collections such as structured or unstructured interviews, or the use of diaries, or other form of documentary methods? Either with observation alone or with other methods, the researcher using a qualitative approach should have produced, 'thick' or 'rich' data. Does this enhance credibility so it almost feels as if you are there?

When it comes to analysis, does the researcher leave a decision trail so that you can audit the way they have moved through the data collection to the establishment of the categories used to present the findings? Overall, does the researcher convince you that they have tried to be as rigorous as possible throughout the study?

Key Points

- ◆ Observation can be used to produce quantitative or qualitative data.

- ◆ Although it is not used as often as some of the other methods, it can play an important part in answering important questions in a holistic and woman-centred way.

- ◆ In observation the main issue is the extent to which the researcher can control the influence of their presence on what is observed.

- ◆ There are a large number of decisions to make prior to the study by the researcher. These include the nature of the role they will play, the amount of interaction they will have with those observed, the method of recording, the extent of recording, and the method of analysis.

- ◆ The time period needed for some studies makes this a costly method of collecting data, and one that requires a large amount of personal skills, as well as research expertise. The benefits of such an approach, however, are considerable.

References

Brink P and Wood M (1994) Basic Steps in Planning Nursing Research (4th edn). Boston: Jones and Bartlett.

Burns N and Grove S (2001) The Practice of Nursing Research: Conduct, Critique, and Utilization (4th edn). Philadelphia: W.B. Saunders.

Davies R (1996) Practitioners in their own right: an ethnographic study of the perceptions of student midwives. In: Robinson S and Thomson A (eds) Midwives, Research and Childbirth. Volume 4. London: Chapman and Hall.

DePoy E and Gitlin L (1994) Introduction to Research: Multiple Strategies for Health and Human Services. St Louis: Mosby.

Holloway I and Wheeler S (1996) Qualitative Research for Nurses. Oxford: Blackwell.

Hunt S and Symonds A (1995) The Social Meaning of Midwifery. Houndmills: Macmillan.

Kirham M (1989) Midwives and information-giving during labour. In: Robinson S and Thomson A (eds) Midwives, Research and Childbirth. Volume 1. London: Chapman and Hall.

LoBiondo-Wood G and Haber J (2002) Nursing Research: Methods, Critical Appraisal, and Utilization (5th edn). St Louis: Mosby.

Morse J and Field P (1996) Nursing Research: The Application of Qualitative Approaches (2nd edn). London: Chapman and Hall.

Phillips R (1996) Observation as a method of data collection in qualitative research. British Journal of Midwifery 4(1): 22, 35–39.

Polit D, Beck B and Hungler B (2001) Essentials of Nursing Research: Methods, Appraisal, and Utilization (5th edn). Philadelphia: Lippincott.

Richens Y (2002) Are midwives using research evidence in practice? British Journal of Midwifery 10(1): 11–16.

Streubert H and Carpenter D (1999) Qualitative Research in Nursing: Advancing the Humanistic Imperative (2nd edn). Philadelphia: Lippincott.

UKCC (1998) Midwives Rules and Code of Practice. London: UKCC.

CHAPTER TWELVE

Experiments

The prominence of clinical effectiveness has increased the demand for research that can unambiguously demonstrate the best options for treatment and care. Experimental design has established itself as the most widely recognized, and respected approach to achieving this evidence. In medicine, the most popular form of the experiment is the randomized control trial (RCT). This method of collecting research data has become so powerful in determining the effectiveness of treatments, that it is used by some as a measure against which all other methods are compared.

The basic goal of the experiment is to produce overwhelming evidence of the existence of a cause and effect relationship between two variables. These are the independent variable (the cause), and the dependent variable (the effect). In medicine this takes the form of the treatment or intervention such as a drug or surgery, and an increase in recovery or level of health (however measured) as the clinical outcome. Such studies usually take the form of a comparison in outcomes between an experimental and control group: the former receiving the drug or intervention, and the latter receiving either the usual treatment or a placebo.

As many clinical procedures in maternity care are influenced by both midwifery and obstetric experimental research, it is crucial that midwives are able to evaluate such studies and not accept them without question. However, one problem is that the presentation of such studies is dominated by the statistical analysis of the data. This can form a barrier to comprehension. Midwives can become depowered if they do not understand the language and conventions of clinical trails, and know how to interpret the findings. Similarly, midwives should know how to carry out relevant trials alone, or as an informed partner in multidisciplinary trails.

The purpose of this chapter is to consider the basic principles of experimental design, and to recognize the strengths, as well as the limitations of this approach. As experiments cover a wide range of designs, the chapter will also outline some of their alternative forms.

Why are experiments special?

Experiments are sometimes regarded not only as different from other broad research approaches such as surveys, but also as having a higher status. This may be due to their association with a 'scientific' approach to research that is somehow related to high levels of accuracy. Oakley (1992) also notes that the randomized control trial (RCT) has been characterized within medicine and health care research generally as 'the most scientifically valid method' of research. Some midwifery research texts also give a high prominence to the experimental approach (Hicks 1996).

Why do experimental designs have such a high status, especially amongst the medical community? The answer lies in what they can achieve and the characteristics they possess. Firstly, in terms of what they can achieve, Polit et al (2001) suggest that it is the most powerful design for testing cause and effect relationships for the following reason:

> Because of its special controlling properties, an experiment offers greater corroboration than any other research approach that the independent variable (e.g. diet, drug dosage, teaching approach) affects the dependent variable (e.g., weight loss, recovery of health, learning).
> (p. 174)

The confirmation of a cause and effect relationship is provided by a statistical calculation of the extent to which the results could have happened by chance. This is indicated by the 'P' value that is frequently to be found in or under a table of results, or in the text of a research article. It is reasonably easy to interpret this, once you are familiar with the basic idea underpinning probability (see Box 12.1).

Characteristics of experimental design

What are the essential features of an experiment? According to LoBiondo-Wood and Haber (2002), the three elements that confirm a study as a true experiment are:

◆ Randomization
◆ Manipulation
◆ Control.

Together these three elements help to rule out competing ways of explaining a particular outcome to a study other than the one proposed by the researcher. Each of these will now be examined in turn.

Randomization

Randomization is a term that may apply to both the sampling procedure used in a study, and the allocation of individuals to a control or intervention group. Random sampling occurs when every member of a study population (all those with the relevant characteristics) has an equal chance of being included in the study. This is not easy to achieve, as individuals must first agree to take part in a clinical study; it is not simply a case of picking them out of a population and expecting them to accept the form of intervention allocated to them. In most cases randomization refers to *random assignment* or *random allocation*. This is the process of allocating participants who have agreed to take part in a study in either the experimental or control group in a random manner. In other words, an individual entering the study should have an equal chance of receiving the treatment or intervention.

The implication of not using random allocation is that there is a risk of developing groups that initially differ from each other. This would make it impossible to rule out the influence of other factors, or independent

Probability values indicate the extent to which the difference in the results between two groups could have happened by chance. The 'P' stands for '*probability*'. This translates into how many times out of a hundred, or even a thousand, the difference between two groups of data could happen purely by chance. The smaller the likelihood that a difference could have happened by chance, the more certain we can be that the experiment has demonstrated a cause and effect situation. In other words, the intervention does produce the desired effect.

The value of 'P' is expressed as a decimal, and has to be converted to a fraction to work out the element of chance. Take the example of '$P < 0.05$'. We first of all convert 0.05 to a fraction by drawing a line underneath the figure; putting a '1' underneath the decimal point, and a '0' underneath every figure after the point. This may sound complicated, but if you write it out for yourself, 0.05 becomes 5/100. In other words the likelihood of the difference between the results of two groups in the study happening purely by chance is less than 5 in 100 times. Or, put another way, 95 times out of 100 the effect you wanted will be produced by the intervention used in the study.

This figure of $P < 0.05$ is regarded as the minimum value that may suggest a relationship between the dependent and independent variable. Notice that there is still a margin of error. It does not mean that one thing definitely causes the other; the results would have happened purely by chance 5 in 100 times. This means that for 95% of the time you can be satisfied that a cause and effect relationship does exist.

The most frequently used values to indicate probability are as follows:

P value	Probability of difference happening by chance
<0.05	less than 5 in 100
<0.01	less than 1 in 100
<0.001	less than 1 in 1000
NS	non-significant (i.e. the probability that chance is responsible for the result is so large that a 'P' value is not used).

It is recommended that you consult a statistics book such as Clegg (1982) for more information.

Box 12.1 Probability values

variables, on the dependent variable at the close of a study. The generalization of the results to other situations would then be very difficult. Where randomization has been achieved it reduces the influence of researcher bias. This is because the researcher is unable to manipulate the results by carefully choosing the experimental group in such a way as to produce the desired outcome. Randomization also ensures that additional factors that may also influence the results are evenly distributed between the two groups. In other words, randomization should allow the researcher to compare like with like.

The existence of a comparison group that does not receive the independent variable is crucial to experimental design. The role of the control group is to act as a comparison by establishing what the typical outcome would be without the influence of the experimental variable. The control group theoretically remains the same over the experimental period, as they do not receive the treatment or intervention that forms the independent variable. This allows the investigator to reduce the effect of what has variously been referred to as the *'attention factor'*, or the *'Hawthorne effect'*. These terms relate to a phenomenon where individuals may experience change simply through participation in a study. In other words, a change in the dependent variable may be due to a feeling of being 'special' that produces a reaction that 'mimics' a real change. In other words there might be apparent change but it would not be produced by the intervention.

Not all studies have a separate group forming the control. One group can receive two interventions in turn, for example, a conventional approach followed by an experimental approach. In this way individuals act as their own control. It is also possible for two separate groups to receive the same two interventions, but in a different order. Here again they are acting as their own controls in that they receive both interventions and rule out the possibility that any differences are the result of varying characteristics of those in the two groups. This kind of approach is referred to as a *cross-over study*.

Manipulation

Experimental designs differ from descriptive research in that the researcher actively does something to some of those in a study. They do not simply record what is happening, but intervene in processes of care to make a difference, one that hopefully will be of benefit to those involved. This is the nature of manipulation. Cluett and Bluff (2000) define the term by saying it is the purposeful introduction of some form of intervention.

Hicks (1996) suggests that the simplest way to find out whether a relationship exists between two variables is to alter one and see what difference it makes to the other. It is the researcher's ability to apply and withhold the independent variable that is unique to the true experiment. Manipulation, then, helps to verify that the outcome is due to the independent variable and not something else.

Control

Under control, the researcher must try to reduce the possible effect of other independent variables on the outcome. This means that the experimenter must have the ability to not only control the independent variable but also other elements within the experimental setting that might make a difference to the outcome. For example, they must be able to choose who takes part in the study, or at least ensure that everyone in the study has an equal chance of being in the experimental group (random allocation). If this is achieved then the researcher can say that they have controlled for extraneous factors that may influence the dependent variable.

It is the researcher's ability to achieve maximum control that illustrates the degree of rigour in the study. This includes control over the way any interventions are provided. All procedures must be applied in exactly the same way to each individual. Measurements of the dependent variable should also be under the control of the researcher. The measuring instrument should be accurate and consistent, and where more than one person is involved in the measurement, the researcher should ensure that everyone is measuring in the same way. This is called inter-rater reliability.

Blinding

There are two important aspects of control that need to be highlighted as they are becoming more important in assessing the rigour of experimental designs. These are *allocation concealment* and *blinding*. At the start of a study as individuals are being allocated to the experimental or control group, it is essential that those carrying out the allocation do not know to which group the next person will be allocated. This is because, as Schulz (2001) notes, researchers or those involved in a study have been known to change who gets allocated to which group. This makes comparisons no longer free from bias. Using sealed opaque envelopes so that it is not possible to anticipate the allocation until the envelope has been opened frequently avoids this problem.

Blinding is more complicated and involves more people as the risk of bias can come from several sources. It involves the risk of people acting differently if they know to which group the individual has been allocated during the course of the study. Schultz (2001) provides a clear explanation of this as follows:

> Blinding or masking involves keeping patients, clinicians, outcome assessors, and /or data analysts unaware of patient allocation to avoid bias. For example, if unblinded, patients may have a heightened sensitivity to the good (or bad) effects of the treatment, clinicians may unwittingly alter the way they provide care or look for a good or adverse outcomes, outcome assessors may distort outcome measurement, and data analysts may alter their approach to analysing the data. Ideally, although not usually possible in studies evaluating nursing intervention, all 4 groups are blinded.
> (p. 5)

Single blinding is where either the person receiving an intervention, or the person measuring the outcome is shielded from knowing whether the experimental intervention or the control has been given. Double blinding is where both the study individual and those measuring the outcome are unaware of the group to which the individual was allocated. As Schultz (2001) points out, double blinding perhaps wrongly, suggests the involvement of two parties, when in reality more than two can be involved. These typically include the individual in the study, the clinician, and the person measuring outcomes.

Taken together, the two aspects of allocation concealment and blinding are amongst the most important aspects of RCTs, as they can have a drastic effect on the accuracy of the outcome. Schultz (2001) suggests that the researcher must not only pay attention to these aspects, but also ensure that the written report clearly demonstrates to the reader that these elements have been carried out to a high standard. According to Schultz, allocation concealment is more important than blinding. He also makes an important point that where trials cannot be double blinded, as is the case in midwifery research, they must be judged on other merits and not that of an inappropriate standard, based on double blinding. This is certainly the case in midwifery research, as in nursing, where the intervention may not be as easily disguised or counterfeited as in medical research.

The hypothesis

Brink and Wood (1994) categorize the experiment as a level three research question (see Chapter 2). To achieve this level they suggest that the researcher should be able to predict what will happen (have a hypothesis), and provide a theory based on previous research findings to explain it. One of the chief purposes of the experiment then, is to test a hypothesis and so establish causality. The researcher should state the hypothesis at the start of the study. This statement can take two forms: the *scientific hypothesis* and the *null-hypothesis*. The scientific hypothesis states the predicted difference in outcomes between the two groups. It usually contains words such as *'more than'* or *'less than'*. The null-hypothesis predicts that there will be no difference between the two groups (see Chapter 7).

For those unfamiliar with hypotheses, it is not always easy to work out which is the dependent and which is the independent variable in the statement. One helpful method of distinguishing between the two is to identify which comes first chronologically and which comes last. The item that comes last is the dependent variable (the effect), and the item that comes first is the independent variable (the cause). Box 12.2 provides some examples of hypotheses and illustrates the dependent and independent variables in each case.

In each of the examples below, identify what chronologically would have to be measured first. This will be the independent variable; the last item to be measured will be the dependent variable.

♦ Length of postnatal hospital stay (*independent variable*) directly affects breastfeeding rates at one month (*dependent variable*) (Winterburn and Fraser 2000).

♦ The use of a new device (maternity gel pad) (*independent variable*) is more effective at reducing levels of perineal oedema, (*dependent variable*), bruising (*dependent variable*), and pain (*dependent variable*) in post-delivered women, following an instrumental delivery when compared with standard regimes (ice packs and Epifoam) (*independent variables*) at the study hospital (Steen et al 2000).

♦ The treatment of women under 37 weeks pregnant with idiopathic preterm labour or prelabour rupture of the membranes with oral broad-spectrum antibiotics (Augmentin and erythromycin) (*independent variable*) reduces the neonatal morbidity (*dependent variable*) associated with preterm birth (Kenyon and Taylor 1995).

Box 12.2   Examples of scientific hypotheses

Types of experiments

Medical research is frequently associated with the RCT. As a method it is still relatively young, being just over fifty years old. Oakley (1992) traces its origins to the work of the Medical Research Council (MRC) and the introduction of streptomycin as a treatment for TB. Studies of the drug, as is now usual (Cross and Nears 2000), were first carried out on animals and these suggested the drug might be an effective cure for the disease. The animals subjected to the test were guinea pigs, hence the expression 'to be a guinea pig', meaning the subject of an experiment. As there was a shortage of the new drug streptomycin, and a large number of people with TB, the MRC allocated what supplies they had on the basis of random selection, using a table of random numbers. The outcome was then monitored in those receiving the drug and a control group, in an attempt to confirm the effectiveness of the drug on humans with TB. This was the first documented use of the RCT.

Experimental design can take a number of alternative forms. The classic writers on the subject, Campbell and Stanley (1963), suggest that there are three main variations:

◆ The pre-test post-test control group

◆ The post-test only design

◆ The Solomon four-group design.

The pre-test post-test control group

This is perhaps the most well known design where subjects are randomly allocated to the experimental or control group. Both groups are observed prior to any intervention, and this acts as a base-line measurement. Any important differences between the two groups should be minimal. In the intervention phase, the experimental group receives the new intervention, whilst the control group receives either the current, or no treatment (although they may receive a placebo). Following a course of treatment, both groups are retested, and any differences subjected to statistical analysis. This calculates the possibility that differences could be due to chance, and not the result of the experimental intervention (Fig. 12.1).

This method can be carried out using two different groups measured over the same time period, or a single group using a cross-over design. This allows those in the study to act as their own controls. The advantage is that it reduces the possibility that those in the two groups are not alike and so do not form true comparisons. Hicks (1996) calls the first approach using two different groups *unrelated, between,* or *different subject* designs, and the second a *related, within* or *same subject* design. It is worth considering that where one group receives both interventions, there can be a 'carry-over' effect, where benefits from the first treatment may still influence the individual once exposed to the second intervention. To reduce this possibility, the order of the interventions is sometimes randomized.

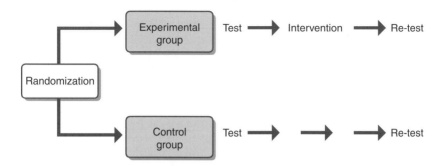

Fig. 12.1 The pre-test, post-test design

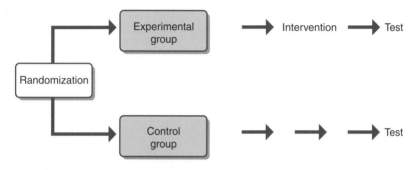

Fig. 12.2 The post-test only design test

Post-test only design

A problem with the pre-test post-test design is that measuring the groups before treatment is not always possible. There is also the problem that the first measurement may sensitize the subjects in such a way that they perform better on the second occasion because of the experience gained from the first measurement. The post-test only design (Fig. 12.2) is an attempt to reduce this familiarity effect by only measuring the variables at the end of the experimental period. The limitation of this design is that it is not possible to say whether the two groups were similar at the start of the study. The difference in measurement could have been due to characteristics existing within the groups before the intervention.

Solomon four-group design

In order to overcome the disadvantages of both the previous examples, the Solomon four-group design has been developed. As can be seen from Figure 12.3, this is really a combination of both the previous designs. This means that as well as being able to eliminate the disadvantage of an after-only design, the effect of pre-testing can be assessed.

The immediate problem is one of gaining a sufficient number of people for all four groups. In addition, the possibility of some people dropping out

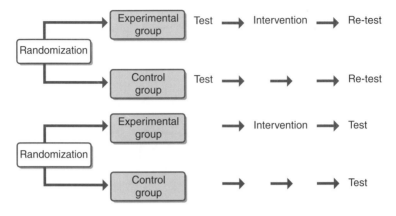

Fig. 12.3 The Solomon four-group design

(subject mortality) is even greater with this number of participants. The researcher may no longer be comparing like with like if the numbers in some of the groups have changed during the study period. This kind of design is very complex to organize and costly. Overall, we can see that this is a large-scale design that requires a great deal of time, resources and expertise.

Threats to validity

Although experimental designs are held in high regard, their use does not guarantee accuracy. There are a number of reasons why the results of an experiment may be inaccurate. Campbell and Stanley (1963) provide the best summary of these problems, usually referred to as threats to validity. These come in two types; those that relate to the experiment itself (*internal threats to validity*) and those that relate to generalizing the results to other situations (*external threats to validity*).

According to Campbell and Stanley (1963), any of the following may result in the researcher incorrectly suggesting they have found a causal relationship between the dependent and independent variable:

◆ *History* (the effect of external events on study outcomes).

In this situation it is not the study's independent variable that has influenced the outcome, but something outside the study, sometimes referred to as a *confounding variable*. For example, media reports highlighting an issue such as problems related to the contraceptive pill, or publicity given to a celebrity choosing to have an elective caesarian section may influence the behaviour, attitude or knowledge of those in a study. The impact of history may be mistaken for the influence (or lack of influence) of an intervention tested in a study.

◆ *Testing* (the effect that being observed or tested has on the study outcomes).

This refers to the consequence of pre-testing, on the results of a later retest. The first test may encourage an individual to think about issues that influence how they answer later in the post-test. Here, it is the influence of the first test and not the intervention that has made a difference to the results.

◆ *Instrumentation* (the extent to which the instrument used to gather information in the study is accurate).

Instrumentation is where pre- and post-differences are due to the data collection instrument changing over time, or the skills or accuracy of the data gatherers changing over time. This may produce different results that are mistakenly interpreted as due to the independent variable.

◆ *Maturation* (the effect of the passage of time on individuals in the sample).

This relates to normal physical, psychological, and social changes that occur to individuals, that are unrelated to the variables in the study. Over time people physically change, adapt, develop new skills, change attitude and so on. This may result in a change between pre- and post-testing results. Maturation changes can also occur over shorter periods. Even in the course of a day we can change physically, or develop insights that if subjected to retesting, may suggest a change due to an intervention rather than a normally occurring event.

◆ *Regression* (a statistical phenomenon).

This is a frequently observed situation in statistics where there is a tendency for extreme scores or measurements in a study to move closer to the mean (average) when repeated testing takes place. This relates to before and after measurements (pre-test/post-test).

◆ *Mortality* (the effect caused by people dropping out of a study before all the measurements have been made).

Although an experimental and control group may have been similar at the start of a study, those who decided to drop out of a study may share common characteristic such as age, parity, or smokers, etc. Those remaining are no longer quite as similar as those in the other group, so the researcher is no longer comparing like with like.

◆ *Interactive effects* (the extent to which each of these threats interact to influence the outcome of a study).

In the same way that the individual threats may influence those in one group rather than another, so the range of influences may be acting on all those selected and so influence the results.

External validity considers those factors that limit the extent to which findings can apply to other settings. There are three main threats that need to be considered, and these relate to i) the people selected for inclusion in the study; ii) the factors relating to what happens within the experiment itself, and iii) the measurements carried out to produce the results.

LoBiondo-Wood and Haber (2002) refer to these as:

◆ Selection effects
◆ Reactive effects
◆ Measurement effects.

Selection effects relates to the extent to which the characteristics of the sample may not have been truly representative of the population, and so it is unwise to generalize from the results of this particular sample. For instance, in some experiments women from a particular social class, age group, or parity may have been over-represented in the sample. This may have produced results that cannot be applied to all women.

The *reactive effect* is the way in which some people respond to being in an experimental situation. They may respond in ways that are influenced by feeling special, or by a desire to help the experimenter succeed or have positive results. In this situation the results are not really due to the independent variable.

This was found in a classic American study on motivation that looked at people working in the Hawthorne plant of an electricity company in Chicago. Although the study set out to examine the effect of heating and lighting and other environmental factors on output, it was found that whether these factors were raised or lowered, productivity increased. It was realized that it was not the heating or lighting affecting the output, but feeling special because they were receiving attention from the researchers that influenced their work level. This gave rise to the term 'Hawthorne effect', mentioned earlier in this chapter, which relates to the reactive effect of being part of a study.

Finally, the *measurement effect* considers the effect of testing on those in a study. If we accept that pre-testing knowledge or attitude may influence retesting, (due to people having an opportunity to reflect on how they feel about the subject of the test), then we have to acknowledge that testing may reduce the extent to which the results of the study can be applied to others. This is because following testing, those in the sample are no longer typical of other people, as they have experienced something, or reflected on subjects or values that now makes them different from others who have not been so exposed.

One further problem area relates to the experimenter. Bias may develop where the researcher in their enthusiasm for the study may subconsciously influence people in non-verbal ways, such as positive nods of the head, or smiling when certain answers are given. This source of error has been described as the experimenter bias effect (Hicks 1996). Similarly, those in the study may provide answers or try hard to carry out the wishes of the experimenter because they like the individual and want the study to be successful. Their reactions to the procedures may also be affected by their knowledge of whether they are in the experimental or control group.

These problems can be tackled by means of blind and double blind studies, discussed above.

Quasi-experimental and ex post facto designs

Although experimental design is regarded as one of the strongest methods of establishing cause and effect relationships, it is not always possible to use this approach in every situation. The reasons for this can be practical, such as difficulties in controlling the effect of other independent variables, or ethical, where it would not be acceptable to allocate people to an experimental and control group. For example, it would not be ethical to allocate some women to say a caesarian section group or normal delivery group, as this would take away choice. Similarly, it would not be possible to randomly allocate women to a smoking or non-smoking group to examine the consequence of smoking on the fetus.

Where it is not possible to meet the strict conditions of experiments, there are a number of near alternatives that can be used. The *quasi-experiment* is one such option. This looks very much like an experiment with often an experimental and control group, and with the researcher introducing an intervention. It differs from a true experiment because is lacks either control, or randomization. In most cases it is the lack of random allocation to the two groups that is missing. An example would be women on one ward having sessions on relaxation to measure its effect on mood and a positive attitude to coping with life following delivery, and those on a second ward being used as a control without relaxation. This makes management of the research easier, as all those in one setting will receive the same approach. It also reduces the risk of 'contamination' where individuals may be influenced by what they see happening to those alongside them.

Unfortunately, having all those in one setting receiving the intervention, rather than random allocation, will weaken the extent to which we have compared like with like. Differences between those in the two groups could make a difference to the outcome. In the relaxation example, it could be that some women already practice yoga, or meditation, or there could be differences in personality between women on the two wards.

For this reason quasi-experimental studies are not as persuasive as a true experimental design. It is possible to strengthen them by taking measurements of both groups prior to the intervention so that we can see the extent to which they are similar and can be accepted as reasonably comparable. In research terms, this approach of two non-randomized groups is referred to as non-equivalent control group design.

Ex post facto studies

In quasi-experimental design, although randomization was not achieved, the researcher still manipulated the independent variable, exposing the experimental group to the intervention, but not the control group. In some situations, not only is it difficult to carry out randomization, but it can also be difficult to manipulate the independent variable. In this instance the solution is the use of an *ex post facto* study. This term means that the difference between the two groups in relation to the independent variable has already happened ('ex post facto' means *'after the fact'*). So, for instance, we might be interested in establishing whether going to antenatal classes has some bearing on the successful use of birth plans. It would be difficult to construct a study and allocate women to the antenatal class attendance group, and others to the antenatal class non-attendance group, as it would mean withholding access to facilities to some people who might want to attend classes and for whom they would be beneficial.

An ex post facto study would collect data on women who were judged to have made good use of a birth plan and those who made little use of a birth plan, and try to establish if there was any pattern as to which group had the highest level of attendance at antenatal classes. In this design we are looking for associations provided by correlation. This statistical process allows us to identify the extent to which factors seem to go together. Unfortunately, we cannot say that one causes the other, only that they appear to be linked. However, this may be satisfactory in providing the basis for midwifery action, or increasing our ability to predict certain events.

The strength of both quasi-experimental and ex post facto designs is their practical nature. They are far more feasible and because they avoid some of the ethical issues of experimental designs they are very attractive designs for midwifery research.

Conducting research

In deciding to undertake an experimental study, it is important to confirm that this is an appropriate approach. Where the purpose of the study is to determine the existence of a cause and effect relationship, then an experimental approach is the method of choice. If the purpose is to search for factors that are associated with each other, and not necessarily as part of a cause and effect relationship, a correlation design will be more appropriate.

Once the appropriateness of an experimental design has been established, the researcher should ensure that the three defining factors of an experiment are feasible. These are:

◆   Randomization

◆   Manipulation

◆   Control.

In addition to these, the researcher must consider the ethical elements of the study, particularly in relation to possible harm through an intervention, or the withholding of accepted interventions. The research should also avoid raising the expectations of those involved or put them into stressful situations. It is advisable to consult Chapter 8 on ethics to ensure that possible problem areas have been anticipated.

As informed consent is an integral part of experimental approaches, a written consent form for those involved in the study to sign will need to be designed, along with an information sheet. These should be included with your research proposal for the Research Ethics Committee (REC). Examples of these may be available locally from others who have undertaken research, from dissertations in educational libraries, or from the ethics committee itself.

In planning the study, previous research should be examined carefully, with special attention paid to the design. In particular, how did the researchers address the threats to internal and external validity? The literature should also provide clues as to the relevant independent variables to be included, and the additional variables that may confound the results, that is cloud the ability to say that the results have been produced by the independent variable(s) manipulated in the study.

In an experimental study the construction of the hypothesis is a major part of the planning process. This should be a clear statement that includes the dependent and independent variable(s). The form of the hypothesis should be considered in terms of whether it will be directional, that is, it will predict the results of the experimental group will be higher or lower than the control group (referred to as a *one-tailed hypothesis*), non directional, that is, it will suggest there will be a difference without saying whether it will be higher or lower in a particular group (referred to as a *two-tailed hypothesis* as the results could go either way), or a *null-hypothesis*, where it would be stated that there would be no difference between the two groups (see Chapter 7).

It is at this stage serious thought should be given to what information will need to be collected to test the hypothesis. This will have to be in a numeric form, and will be subjected to a statistical test. There are a variety of tests, depending on the form of the experiment and the nature of the numeric values (see Chapter 13). It is at the early design stage that the statistical procedures required should be explored. It is recommended that an appropriate book that includes statistical testing is consulted (e.g. Hicks 1996, Martin and Thomson 2000) and help and advice sought from someone who is knowledgeable in statistical techniques.

In order to reduce bias as much as possible, thought needs to be given as to who will collect the data. In some instances it may be feasible, as well as highly desirable, to have someone not directly involved with the design of the study collect data blind, that is, without knowing the hypotheses to be tested, and without knowing whether subjects are in the experimental or control group. At the design stage the necessity and method of blinding the subjects should also be considered to produce a double blind study. Remember that in midwifery, it is not always realistic to expect that those in the study will not know what intervention they have received.

Where several people are collecting data, steps should be taken to ensure they measure, code, or collect the information in exactly the same way and with the same degree of accuracy (referred to as *inter-rater* or *inter-observer reliability*). This attention to consistency and accuracy should extend to any equipment used as part of the study, or any materials such as Likert scales or other form of measurements.

The way the study is carried out must be carefully recorded in sufficient detail so that it can be used by anyone wishing to replicate the study. A pilot study is essential to familiarize them with the equipment and the procedure.

When conducting the main study, the safety and welfare of the subjects is paramount. In some instances the decision may have to be made to immediately remove individuals from the study for their own benefit, and transfer them to standard procedures, or treatments. On other occasions, there may be factors that develop during the study that make some people no longer typical within the group, and they may have to be excluded at the analysis stage. All these factors relate to the rigour of the study.

At the end of an experimental study it is important to base the conclusions only on the results. The statistical tests will provide some answer as to the strength of the relationship between the independent and dependent variables. It is important to recognize that these tests only relate to a statistical relationship between the figures and do not necessarily imply that a real world relationship exists. There is always a margin of error in experimental studies. In addition, the sometimes artificial circumstances and environment of an experiment can make generalizations difficult. Medicine has always placed a great emphasis on replication studies to ensure that the results of a single study do not influence practice without the corroboration of further studies. It is important that midwifery also recognizes the importance of replication studies.

Where it is not possible for practical or ethical reasons to carry out a true experimental design, then the researcher should choose the next appropriate design, such as quasi-experimental or ex post facto designs. These may play an important part in providing valuable answers for practice. The rigour of these designs is just as important as in experimental designs, if not more so. This is because an evaluation of such studies will start with the view that they are not as strong as experimental design. Clear attempts should therefore be made to reduce the possibility of the results being explained by factors other than the ones being suggested by the researcher.

All the designs in this section depend on a very clear statistical presentation of the results. It is this aspect of research reports that many midwives find most demanding. For this reason the midwifery researcher should explain the statistical procedures used, and clarify their meaning and implications for the reader as clearly as possible.

Critiquing research

Critiquing experimental research can be challenging, mainly because of the reader's unfamiliarity with statistical presentation. Yet a little knowledge and understanding of some of the basic concepts and conventions can clarify the report drastically (see Chapter 13). The first stage of critiquing is to ensure that the researcher is searching for a cause and effect relationship between an independent and dependent variable. This will usually be evident from the wording of the terms of reference that will suggest the influence of one variable on another. Experimental research should contain a hypothesis, although sadly, this is not present in all reports.

In examining the details of the conduct of the study the three features of an experiment, manipulation, control and randomization, should be present. If randomization, or control is not present, it may be a quasi-experimental study. Again few studies state they are using this as the design. If the researcher states the intention is to look for associations or possible relationships, then the study is likely to be a correlation design. Here it will not be possible for the researcher to talk in terms of cause and effect, or dependent and independent variables.

Where the study is clearly experimental, consideration should be given to the ethical component. Was the study approved by an ethics committee, or in the case of an American article, an Institutional Review Board (IRB)? To what extent did those in the study clearly give their informed consent? Was it made clear that participation in the study was optional, and it was possible to withdraw at any point? Did the author assess possible harm, and build in safeguards to discontinue involvement or, through clear exclusion criteria, prevent any vulnerable individuals from entering the study in the first place? Although all these questions are important, not all articles will provide answers to these aspects of the study.

The sample included in the study should be scrutinized in relation to the inclusion and exclusion criteria for those selected for the study. The method of randomization should be examined to ensure that everyone had an equal chance of being selected for the experimental group. A close comparison should then be made of the groups to ensure that they are comparable in those factors that might have made a difference to the results. Remember they should be as similar as possible in all respects apart from the exposure to the independent variable under study.

The researcher should give clear concept and operational definitions for the dependent and independent variables. These should be considered for their adequacy. The type of intervention should be considered carefully in terms of how did the researcher make sure that it was provided in a similar way to everyone? Was there a check on this, such as training for those involved in providing the intervention to ensure consistency? In particular, an assessment should be made of possible inaccuracies in the measurements made following the intervention. Was this a blind or double blind study? If either of these is used, are details provided of how this was achieved? If there was no blinding, does this suggest any possible weaknesses?

In examining the results section, has the researcher used an appropriate test of significance to test the probability that any differences between groups could have happened by chance? Here the size of the 'P' value is important. In considering the results, to what extent has the researcher taken into account the possible threats to internal and external validity? It is worth considering whether the results could be explained by some other factor besides the independent variable.

Depending on the results, what are the implications for practice? What specific recommendations are made in the report? Whatever the researcher says, it is important to remember the importance of the reliability of the data collection tool(s), the validity of the study in terms of is there evidence that they have measured what they believe they have measured? Are there any biasing factors concerning those selected for the study? And finally, are you satisfied with the rigour with which the researcher conducted the study? Is there a striving for excellence in the way the whole study was designed and carried out?

Above all, do not simply be impressed by the size of the study, its complexity, or the use of statistics. As with any kind of study, it is crucial to challenge the research. Consider both the researcher's attempts to maintain accuracy and the limitations of their study. These will have implications for the extent to which you can generalize the results to your own situation. With all clinical trials, it is wise to look for confirmation from replication studies before adopting a system that may have considerable implications for individual safety and quality of care.

Key Points

♦ Experimental designs, particularly in the form of the randomized control trial, have become one of the most respected types of research in the health service. The reason for this relates to the way that drugs and treatments in the past have been carefully tested to reduce the possibility of other explanations for the results.

♦ The conduct of experimental studies can be very complex because they are dependent on the three necessary experimental elements of control, manipulation and randomization. In midwifery, it is not always possible, or desirable, to achieve these elements. Sometimes it would be unethical, or at least drastically reduce women's choice or individual midwife's judgement as to what was best in the particular circumstances, if strict experimental protocols were followed.

♦ There are compromises to a full experimental design available such as quasi-experimental, ex post facto and correlation designs. Although these do not produce conclusions that are as 'strong' as experimental designs, they can still inform evidence-based practice.

♦ Despite the status given to experimental designs, they do have their limitations. It is not always possible to control for other factors that may explain the results. In addition, it is sometimes an over-simplification to look for one cause for a phenomenon; sometimes there are several.

♦ Integral to this type of design is the application of statistical methods, particularly inferential statistics. These identify the influence of chance in explaining the difference in the results between groups. The knowledge required to understand and challenge this form of research is therefore more demanding than some of the other methods. Midwives should not see this as a reason for avoiding using this research approach, or avoid reading published work that centres on its use. The effort needed to gain the statistical knowledge and understanding is well worth the reward of being able to confidently use and challenge this research approach.

References

Brink P and Wood M (1994) Basic Steps in Planning Nursing Research (4th edn). Boston: Jones and Bartlett.

Cambell D and Stanley J (1963) Experimental and Quasi-experimental Design. Chicago: Rand McNally.

Clegg F (1982) Simple Statistics. Cambridge: Cambridge University Press.

Cluett E and Bluff R (2000) Principles and Practice of Research in Midwifery. Edinburgh: Baillière Tindall.

Cross R and Nears A (2000) Clinical trials: a journey of discovery. Nursing Standard 14(39): 44–47.

Hicks C (1996) Undertaking Midwifery Research: A Basic Guide to Design and Analysis. New York: Churchill Livingstone.

Kenyon S and Taylor D (1995) ORACLE study: midwives will play a crucial part. British Journal of Midwifery 3(2): 75–78.

LoBiondo-Wood G and Haber J (2002) Nursing Research: Methods, Critical Appraisal, and Utilization (5th edn). St Louis: Mosby.

Martin C and Thompson D (2000) Design and analysis of Clinical Nursing Research Studies. London: Routledge.

Oakley A (1992) Social Support and Motherhood. Oxford: Blackwell.

Polit D, Beck B and Hungler B (2001) Essentials of Nursing Research: Methods, Appraisal, and Utilization (5th edn). Philadelphia: Lippincott.

Schultz K (2001) Assessing allocation concealment and blinding in randomised controlled trial: why bother? Evidence-Based Nursing 1(4): 4–5.

Steen M, Cooper K, Merchant P, Griffiths-Jones and Walker J (2000) A randomised controlled trial to compare the effectiveness of icepacks and Epifoam with cooling maternity gel pads at alleviating postnatal perineal trauma. Midwifery 16(1): 48–55.

Winterburn S and Fraser R (2000) Does the duration of postnatal stay influence breast-feeding rates at one month in women giving birth for the first time. A randomised control trial. Journal of Advanced Nursing 32(5): 1152–1157.

CHAPTER THIRTEEN
Statistics in Research

This is the chapter you may be tempted to skip, however, don't pass on just yet. Understanding the way numbers are presented in research is one of the most important skills in making sense of research articles. It is also essential if you are to clearly present your own numeric findings. In order to read research papers in greater depth, every midwife needs to understand just a small number of statistical principles. These will play an important role in establishing whether the author's conclusions are justified. So although it is easy to ignore the statistical sections in research, understanding them does have a direct effect on care. Indeed, Cluett (2000) suggests that mastery of statistics enables midwives to offer every woman high quality, women-centred care.

Why, then, are we so fearful of statistics? For many people the figures, signs, and abbreviations may seem like a secret code (Critchton 2001). Perhaps they remind us of unpleasant experiences in school where we felt lost or left behind. For some, the easiest way of coping with these feelings is to give up, and pretend statistics do not matter. They do. The current emphasis on evidence-based practice in health care, and the role of quantitative research in evaluating the outcome of interventions, means we can no longer pretend that a basic understanding of statistics is of no consequence.

For those ready to make a fresh start, this chapter will explain some of the statistical procedures you will meet in many research reports. You will not have to learn how to carry out complicated calculations; there are specialized books and courses that will help you if you need to know this. The aim of the following sections is to explain why various procedures are used; the basic principles underpinning them, and how to interpret them.

If the very word 'statistics' frightens you, let's start by clarifying its meaning. Statistics, according to Diamond and Jefferies (2001) is concerned with understanding and knowing how to use data. Many writers on the subject do appreciate our difficulty with the subject, as some of the titles for beginners show. Take the following:

Statistics For People Who (Think they) Hate Statistics – Salkind (2000)

Statistics From Scratch For Health Care Professionals – Bowers (1996)

Simple statistics – Clegg (1982)

All of these books present their subject in a light-hearted way and emphasize that most statistics are very straightforward; it is just the unfamiliarity of the presentation that can be baffling.

As with research in general, there are some unusual words and symbols to learn and some familiar words that have different meanings (see Table 13.1). One example is the word *'significant'*. This does not mean 'important', but suggests that the difference in the outcomes between two groups in, say, a randomized control trial (RCT), is unlikely to have happened by chance. In other words, the difference between the two groups is more likely to be explained by what the researcher did, than by any other explanation. Similarly, the word '*data*' is plural, so you will see the word '*are*' not '*is*' following it, as well as expressions such as 'the data *were* calculated', not '*was*' calculated.

There is also a common misconception about statistics we should dismiss. It is not true to say '*you can prove anything with statistics*' – rather some people can misuse them, or ignore the rules that affect their use. Most research papers are based on a relatively small number of accepted procedures and assumptions. You do not have to understand exactly how something was calculated, as long as you understand the basic principle underpinning its use and you can 'read' the symbols and statements used by the researcher.

Two types of statistic

There are two major categories of statistic used in research: *descriptive* statistics and *inferential* statistics. Descriptive statistics use numbers to paint a picture of features or variables found in a sample, whilst inferential statistics are used to say something about the features or variables within the wider population from which the sample was taken. Inferential statistics are an essential part of randomized control trials (RCTs) as they indicate the extent to which the intervention introduced by the researcher had an impact on the outcome. They also provide an indication of whether the results from the sample are likely to exist in the wider group or population from which the sample was taken. Inferential statistics also include the use of *correlation*; this indicates a pattern or association between variables, for example, in a survey.

Descriptive statistics

If we get down to basics, quantitative research is concerned with measuring a variable in a way that produces a numeric value. Some variables such as weight; time, amount of fluid lost, etc. have clear operational definitions in the form of standard units of measurement. For some attributes, such as the degree of tear following delivery, or condition of baby at birth, scales have been devised such as the degree of the tear, and Apgar score. Other elements such as satisfaction with the delivery, or the amount of information received on screening procedures, may have to be turned into numeric values. This is achieved using approximate measures such as Likert scales where the individual may be given a number of statements and asked to choose from such options as 'strongly agree', 'agree' etc. The researcher allocates each point on the scale a number such as:

Strongly agree	Agree	Undecided	Disagree	Strongly disagree
5	4	3	2	1

Table 13.1   Common statistical symbols and their meaning

Symbol	Meaning	Use
Σ	Greek symbol meaning add together what follows	As part of a formula providing instructions, e.g. Σx, which means add together each value for the variable collected.
<	Less than	Indicates set value e.g. $P < 0.05$ means that the value of P is below or smaller than 0.05.
>	Greater than	Indicates the opposite of the above as in $P > 0.05$, which means that the value is greater than 0.05. The open end of the symbol means greater than, and the closed end means less than reading from the left hand side of the symbol.
≥	Equal to or greater than	To indicate a condition to be met during a calculation.
±	Plus and minus the figure that follows	Used for example in standard deviation (sd) where the figure that follows the symbol is taken away from the mean and added to the mean to give the range between which the majority of values in the data set will fall.
χ^2	Symbol for the chi-squared test (pronounced 'ki-squared') as in kite	This test indicates the chances that any differences between the groups in the study could have happened by chance. The test is used with 'nominal data' (i.e. falling into one category or another, such as yes or no) and compares the actual results with what might have been expected if there was no difference between the groups.
$P < 0.05$	Used as part of statistical tests to indicate the level of probability of being wrong if a real difference between the groups involved was assumed.	This is the minimum level set for tests of significance to indicate that the results are unlikely to have happened purely by chance. It means you would be wrong 5 times in 100 if you said there was a real difference between the groups involved. Other values showing a progressively better result include $P < 0.01$ (1 in 100), and $P < 0.001$ (1 in 1,000).

NS	Non significant	This abbreviation suggests that there was not a statistical difference between the outcomes of an experimental and control group. Testing has failed to reach the level $P < 0.05$, therefore there is no real difference between the groups concerned.
r_s	The symbol for Spearman's rho (pronounced 'row')	Used to indicate a correlation between two variables measured at least at ordinal level. The strength of this will be somewhere between $+1$ and -1.
r	The symbol for the Pearson Product-moment (usually referred to as Pearson r)	The same as the above only this is used where both variables are measured at either interval or ratio level. This falls into the category of parametric statistics as it indicates features (parameters) of the population from which the sample is taken.
t	The t-test symbol	This parametric test examines the difference in the means of two groups to see if they are statistically different. There are two versions, the t-test for independent samples, i.e. two different groups, and the t-test for matched or paired groups, i.e. the same group before and after an intervention.
CI	Confidence Interval	This is an upper and lower figure between which the value measured in the sample is estimated to lie in the population as a whole.

The basic principle behind all these procedures is to provide the researcher with some form of numeric measurement that can be processed statistically.

From the examples just used, it can be seen that some numbers express quantities that are more accurate than others. Time and volume may be checked and agreed independently as accurate. Other measurements are less accurate or certain, for example blood loss or dilatation of the cervix. This is an important observation, as some researchers will claim a greater degree of objectivity and accuracy for their data than is possible. For some studies, numbers have been produced more as a convenience to allow statistical procedures to take place than as a precise measurement.

Levels of measurement

Following the point made in the last section, we need to know more about how numbers can differ in their accuracy, and how this affects the kind of statements we can make using them. One way to achieve this is through the concept of *levels of measurement*.

All numbers look the same. Basically you can construct any combination of numbers you like using the numeric keys 0 to 9 on a computer or calculator keyboard. In statistical theory, numbers are used to represent different ideas, depending on the type of number being used. One simple, but very important difference is between the levels of measurement. This indicates how the number is being used. Is it being used to convey the quantity of a unit, or is it simply providing a convenient category label?

There are four levels of measurement. This simply means there are four different ways numbers can be used to convey ideas. These are the levels:

1. Nominal level (or Categorical level)

This is the most basic level. It nominates the variable to a particular category that is mutually exclusive (it can only be put into one category). It uses a number to provide a label for that category. So midwives working only in the community may be categorized under the heading '1', and midwives working only in the hospital setting could be categorized as '2', those working in both might be '3'. This means that those in the category '1' are the same or equivalent; it does not mean that it takes two community midwives to make one hospital midwife, it just provides a label that happens to be a number. They could just as easily have been labelled using a letter of the alphabet, as blood groups are, a colour or anything else.

2. Ordinal level

Numbers used in this second category not only label a category but also indicate sequence or rank order. So, people entering a clinical area might be given the sequential numeric values 1, 2, 3, 4, to indicate the order in which they entered that area. This would indicate that number 3 was two behind number 1, and one ahead of number 4. We cannot do much else with the numbers. We do not know how much later each person was behind the one in front. There may have been a split second between numbers 1 and 2 and several hours before number 3 entered and a day before number 4 entered.

The relevance of this category of measurement is that it takes the same form of the numbers used in a Likert scale or Apgar score. Although the parts of the scale can be labelled 1 to 5, as in the case of a Likert scale, there is no indication of the precise distance between each point. The distance between 'agree' and 'strongly agree', may not be the same as that between 'disagree' and 'strongly disagree'. All that we can say is that the numbers indicate sequence or rank order along a continuum.

Both nominal and ordinal levels of measurement form a single sub category in the levels of measurement and are usually both classed as categorical. They both possess very basic properties that are restrictive to the statistician in terms of the statistical procedures that can be carried out on them. The next two categories are far more sophisticated and provide more useful information.

3. *Interval level*

This level produces numbers that indicate sequence, but this time the distance between the different points are uniform. This means that they can be 'averaged', and other procedures carried out on them. Along with the next category, the interval level can be said to be truly numeric in that it measures amounts and does not simply use numbers to indicate categories.

4. *Ratio level*

This is the final, and highest, level of measurement. It is very much like the interval level except for one crucial factor, and that is there is an absolute zero point in the measurement scale below which it is impossible to record a value. Temperature in Fahrenheit or Centigrade is interval level because it is possible to have a minus figure, such as minus three degrees Centigrade. This is because zero in Fahrenheit is an arbitrary point, not an absolute zero. Height, age and weight are all ratio level as it is impossible to have less than a zero amount of any of them.

The importance of the last two levels is that they quantify something, and they are always measured in units of some kind, such as kilograms, hours and minutes, centilitres, etc. It is this property that makes them suitable for statistical procedures in that the other levels of nominal and ordinal do not measure anything but simply categorize using numbers to label the categories, and in the case of ordinal data, place them in sequence. They do not measure the quantity of anything. For this reason, the interval and ratio levels are classed as numeric levels and the nominal and ordinal levels are seen as categorical levels. The key characteristics of these four levels of measurement are summarized below in Table 13.2.

Many of the principles of statistical analysis are based on this categorization system; therefore, its importance to understanding statistics should not be underestimated. In the next section we turn to the problem of making descriptive statistics meaningful to the reader.

Table 13.2 Properties and characteristics of each level of measurement

Level	Properties	Characteristics
Nominal	Most basic of all	Names, categorizes variables
Ordinal	Basic non measurement	Numbers used to categorize into sequence or 'rank order'
Interval	Measures properties of variable	Equal distance between units; no absolute zero. Sophisticated statistical procedures possible
Ratio	Highest level	Absolute zero, equal distance between units. Suited to sophisticated statistical procedures

Summarizing descriptive data: measures of central tendency

One reason for processing data is to make them easier to understand. It also allows the researcher to communicate important points about their results in simple ways. It is no use presenting results in the form of each individual measure for each variable gathered from each person in its original form, such as the following:

Respondent A: 12 2 2 17 2 5 34 23 7 8 64 34 3 2 46 50
Respondent B: 10 3 4 21 3 8 30 15 1 2 57 41 5 4 57 47

It would mean very little as it is not clear to what the numbers relate, and there is no pattern visible that makes sense. The answer is to use summary statistics that allow us to convey meaning by summarizing quite large collections of numbers.

The most successful form of summary statistic is the *measure of central tendency*. This is a clumsy way of saying the number that appears typical, or around the central value found in the entire collection of results (data-set). If you are thinking 'that sounds like the average' you would be right, but in statistics there are a number of different ways of calculating 'the average', each known by a different name.

I) MEAN
This is what we commonly call the 'average'. For instance we might say 'on average I take half an hour to get home', or we might read that 'on average people watch television for two hours a day'. We don't mean that the figure is exact, sometimes it may be more, sometimes in may be less, but when we even things out it is reasonably typical.

It is not difficult to calculate the 'average' or 'mean' of something. If you had to work out the average length of time that ten members of staff in your clinical area had been qualified, you would ask each one how long they had been qualified, add them all up and divide by the total number of people.

Easy! To teach someone the statistical procedure involved in that calculation, the statistician would use a formula that would symbolize the different elements in the calculations and outline the sequence of steps involved. The formula for the procedure to calculate the mean would look like this:

$$\frac{\Sigma X}{N}$$

The symbols stand for the following:

Σ = Add together each of the following
X = The numeric value of the item you are interested in from each person
— = The sign for 'divide by' used in a fraction
N = The total number in the group.

The formula looks baffling, but understanding the symbols, and the sequence in which to carry out the procedures, makes it clearer. This is how even the most complicated formulae work; each symbol is translated into an activity that is carried out in a particular sequence.

It is worth making the point that the mean can only be calculated if the level of data is either interval or ratio; that is, where the numbers reach a numeric level of measurement and are actually measuring something in recognizable units of measurement. It does not work for categorical data such as calculating the average star sign of people in a group where Aquarius = 1, Pisces = 2, etc. Neither does it really work with ordinal data, although you will see an average figure for Likert scale values calculated.

There is one big drawback in using the mean, and that is it is influenced by untypical numbers that are higher or lower than the majority of other numbers in the group or 'data-set'. These are called 'outliers', because when individual results are plotted on a graph, they are the ones that stand out because they are out of line with the main results. We can sometimes be misled by the mean figure for a group of results because there may be a small number of untypical values pulling the mean up or down. This will be illustrated in Box 13.1.

II) MEDIAN
The median is a useful calculation of central tendency, as it is not influenced by extreme values. The median is calculated by taking every single figure in the set of numbers, such as delivery time for 20 women. They are then put in rank order from the shortest to the longest or smallest to the biggest. The median is the value of the unit in the middle of this row or *distribution* of numbers.

Let's take an example to illustrate the advantage of the median over the mean. Imagine nine children have been booked in to a birthday party at a restaurant. Unfortunately, the only information the restaurant has to prepare for the type of party is the name of the person who made the booking. They need to know whether to provide a children's jelly and blancmange type party, or a fairly wild alcoholic affair. The solution is to telephone and ask for the average (mean) age of those attending.

a) Ages of a group of children going to a birthday party

6 6 8 8 9 9 10 11 11

median = 9, mean = 8.6

b) Ages of children plus Grandma and her twin sister Elsie going to a birthday party

6 6 8 8 9 9 10 72 72

median = 9, mean = 22.2

Punch line: The median is a more stable calculation, as outliers (untypical large or small figures) do not influence it; the mean is influenced by outliers and can produce an unrepresentative figure.

Box 13.1　Ages of those attending a restaurant party

If the set of ages (values) in line a) in Box 13.1 above were used to supply the mean, the figure communicated would be 8.6 or corrected up to the nearest whole figure, 9 years. The median could be calculated once each item in the data set had been put in rank order from the smallest to the biggest (which has already been done), by identifying the 'middle' value. This would be the 5th number as there would be four numbers on either side of it. In this example, the median would also be 9 years.

Now what if the two 11 year olds did not want to be associated with the group and decided to back out, leaving Grandma and her twin sister Elsie, both 72, to accompany the children instead? If the restaurant rang up this time to be told the average age in the party was 22.2, or 22 to the nearest whole figure, they may lay on a very alcoholic adult type of birthday party. However, if they had asked for the median, the value would have still been 9, because it is the position in the rank order that is used to calculate the answer not the combined values.

How is the median calculated where there is an even number of items in the data-set, as in the set below?

6 6 8 8 9 9 10 11

The answer is to first identify the midpoint again. This time it would be a line drawn between 8 and 9, as there would be 4 values on each side of the line. Simply adding the values of the numbers either side of the line together and dividing by two would produce the median of 7.5 years. In other words it is the mean of the combined values of the numbers on either side of the line that splits the ranked sequence of numbers into two halves. Draw a line yourself on the page above, or copy the figures on to paper to check this out if it seems hard to follow.

A good way of remembering what is achieved through calculating the median is that it provides a cut-off point along a ranked order of numbers such that half of all the values are below that cut-off point; the median value, and the remaining half are above it.

There is one disadvantage of the median, and that is it becomes very unwieldy to calculate if there is a very large set of values in the set, as each one has to be placed in rank order to locate the middle value.

III) MODE

The final method of calculating an average is the mode. This is the most frequently appearing value in the set.

If we go back to the set of values in b) in Box 13.1 above, and adjust it slightly to make it:

c) Adjusted distribution of ages

6 6 6 8 8 9 9 10 72 72

The mode would be 6, as that is the number that appears the greatest number of times. However, if there were three 6 year olds and three 9 year olds, then there would be two modes, 6 and 9. This is referred to as a *bimodal distribution*. Just to complicate things, if there had been three 8 year olds as well as three 6 year olds and three 9 year olds, it would have been *multimodal*.

You are probably already getting the feeling that this is not a very useful way of saying what is typical in the group, as the mode can change drastically as a result of one number that can shift the mode anywhere in the distribution. This can be confirmed by taking c) above and changing the first and last digit as follows:

d) Final adjustment of ages

6 6 8 8 9 9 10 72 72 72

We have now swung the mode from one end of the line to the other end by just changing one number. This illustrates the point that each statistical calculation has its own special characteristics, and we have to know something about these in order to know when they can be misleading. When painting a picture of what is typical in a group of results, or what is around the middle value, we have to be very careful which method of calculation we choose, as we can alter the result radically by using a different calculation.

Measures of central tendency: the standard deviation

The last section illustrated that the mean is not the most useful method of calculating the value that stands for, or is typical of, the values in the group. The final statistical method in this section allows us to go back to the mean and make it more effective. This is by using the mean in combination with the standard deviation.

The standard deviation (abbreviation 'sd') is a measurement derived by working out the average distance of each item in a data-set from the mean. If we measured 30 women's height the mean might be 5 foot 4 inches. The standard deviation when calculated to establish the mean distance of each woman's height from the overall mean might work out at 3 inches. The value of the standard deviation is then added to the mean (5 foot 4 ins + 3 inches) to give 5 foot 7 inches as an upper value, and is then taken away from the mean 5 foot 4 inches − 3 inches) to give 5 foot 1 inch as a lower value. Where there is an even pattern in the variable concerned (explained in the following section under the heading 'normal distribution') then the majority of people (around 68%) will lie in this range.

The smaller the standard deviation in relation to the mean, the closer all the values will be to it. This would suggest that the mean is reasonably typical of the values in the group. The larger the standard deviation, the more spread out the values will be, as there will be a large variation between the values above and below the mean (the mean plus and minus the standard deviation). This will indicate that the mean is not very helpful in gaining an idea of what is typical in the group.

The standard deviation is also used to identify if the attributes of those in two groups, for example, in an RCT are closely matched, or whether they are different, and if so, how different. This is achieved by comparing the mean and standard deviation in the two groups. We would not expect the results to be identical, but we would want to feel they were reasonably close and that any discrepancies did not suggest clinically significant variations that might make a difference to the interpretation of the results.

An example of the use of the standard deviation in this way is the work by Carter et al (2001) who looked at maternal bowel and/or urinary dysfunction and child development differences in two groups of women 5 years following delivery. One group were those who had a normal delivery (NVD) and the second group had instrumental vaginal deliveries (IVD).

The comparability between the two groups was examined in relation to a number of variables including the length of the second stage of labour, measured in minutes. This is expressed in terms of the mean and the standard deviation for both groups. Table 13.3 presents this one item taken from a large table of factors.

First of all, reading the first column we can see that it contains the row label, which is the result of the second stage of labour. The first pair of brackets tells us that this is measured in minutes (min). The second bracket indicates that the next figure is the mean result for the group followed by the standard deviation. Looking across the row we can see that the standard deviation has been placed in a bracket to prevent it being confused with the mean. Reading across the top line, which outlines the content of the

Table 13.3 Comparability between two groups of women for length of second stage of labour (reproduced with permission from Carter et al 2001)

	Instrumental delivery group (*n* = 228)	Normal delivery group (*n* = 68)	Statistical significance
Second stage of labour (min) (mean) (SD)	79 (59)	43 (34)	$P < 0.001$

columns, we can see that the second column shows those who received an instrumental delivery and this involved 228 women. The letter '*n*' followed by ' = ' indicates the number of items or people in that category.

Looking at the results we can see that there is a considerable difference in the size of the two groups, with 228 in the instrumental deliveries and 68 in the normal group. When we look at the mean length of the second stage of delivery in each group, we can see that instrumental deliveries were on average almost double the length of normal deliveries, which is something we might have expected. The standard deviations are also very different. The average distance of each delivery in the instrumental group away from the mean (either above it or below it) was almost an hour (59 min) whereas in the normal delivery group, it was almost half that, just under half an hour (34 min) on average above or below it. This tells us that the deliveries in the first group were spread out far more than those in the second group, which tended to be around the half hour mark 'on average' from the mean figure given. The last column tells us to what extent this difference could be a chance finding, or is there likely to be a real difference between the two groups (see Box 12.1 in Chapter 12 on experiments for an explanation of '*P*' values).

Normal distribution

In looking at the way individual values are spread around the mean, there is one particular pattern they can take that is important to the statistician, and this is called the *normal distribution*.

Normal distribution is a theoretical concept that has a major influence on a number of important statistical decisions, including those in inferential statistics discussed below. It relates to interval and ratio data and can be outlined as follows. If we were to plot the frequency distribution of characteristics such as height, blood pressure, from a large number of people on a graph they would form a very distinctive shape. This is because in a large sample the numbers of very tall people and the numbers of very short people appear in about the same ratio with the majority of people being fairly close to the mean height. The curve on the graph would look like the outline of a church bell, where the majority of people would be in the mid section and the slope of the curve of the bell shape would come down to the small number of people on either side of the majority who were either very tall or very short (see Figure 13.1).

The distinctive characteristic of such distribution is that the mean, mode and median would all be the same value. This would appear on a graph as one line passing from the very apex of the bell (the tallest point on the curve), to the baseline of the graph. The shape is said to be symmetrical, in that if we were to cut the shape out of the page on which it appeared, and fold it down the mid line formed by the mean, each side would touch perfectly like a mirror image, without any overlaps.

This kind of a shape has a mathematical property whereby if we measure one standard deviation either side of this midline, then the area under the curve bounded by the upper and lower standard deviation lines would

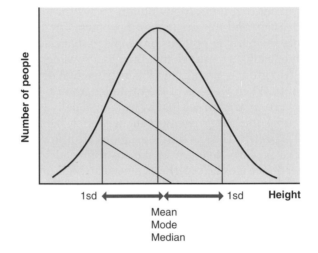

Fig. 13.1   Normal distribution curve showing the height of a group of people

include the values from about 68% of all the individuals in the study. This is a constant result for all variables that have a normal distribution.

The usefulness of this is that if a variable is normally distributed and we know the mean, by calculating the standard deviation and working out one standard deviation above and below the mean, we can be sure that the majority of people in the sample (68%) will measure somewhere between this upper and lower level of measurement. This is shown as:

Mean ± 1 sd

This can be extended to ± 2 sd to give an upper and lower level between which about 95% of all the values will fall. However, most studies use one standard deviation to give a picture of the majority of measurements.

Presentation of descriptive results

Having looked at some of the basic principles of descriptive statistics, we can look at some of the ways results are presented, and how we can make sense of them. Although the researcher will describe the results in the main body or text of their report, they will frequently use some visual displays to help the reader 'see' the results clearer. This visual presentation can take a number of forms, as shown in Table 13.4. These can include summary tables, which present the major numerical findings, and graphical figures such as bar charts, histograms, pie charts and line graphs. Martin and Thompson (2000) emphasize that graphical data presentation is not a substitute for a summary table, which they see as essential in presenting a snap shot of the numerical findings of a study, but is a means of increasing the clarity and accessibility of the results.

Each of these can convey complex information more efficiently than words. The visual presentation means they are uncluttered by descriptions

Table 13.4 Common methods of presenting descriptive data

Type	Description
Tables	Labelled columns and rows of numbers. Can take the form of frequency tables, where just one variable is examined, or cross-tabulations where two or more variables are shown. One variable can then be displayed in terms of another variable, e.g. insufficient information provided to women by trimester on a variety of topics (Lavender et al 2000).
Bar charts	A block diagram used to show amounts of a discrete (can't be broken down into smaller units) variable, such as male/female. The blocks or 'bars' do not touch. They can be shown in a vertical format or horizontal format. They can be 'stacked' bar charts, where each bar totals 100% and is divided into the range of possible sub groups, e.g. responses to the question 'do midwives have a role in a named range of health promotion topics?' (Lavender et al 2001).
Histograms	As above, but shows a continuous (can be broken down into smaller units of measurement) variable. The blocks will touch to show they are on a continuous scale, e.g. histogram showing number of months women continued breastfeeding in one unit following the introduction of the Baby Friendly Initiative (BFI).
Pie charts	This is a circle divided into appropriate 'slices' to show the quantity of different categories. The result must add up to 100%. These work well when there are between three and six slices providing the majority of slices are not too 'thin', e.g. causes of stress felt by midwives (Birch 2001).
Line graph	Lines that join points plotted on a graph to show trends in the data, e.g. percentage of women who indicated they felt prepared for pregnancy, labour and parenthood over a number of time periods (Lavender et al 2000).

and can be located quickly (Cluett 2000). An examination of a visual display also allows the reader to observe the overall pattern or trend of the results, which is more difficult when presented in the form of words. However, the researcher must choose the right format for the information, and the reader must understand the principles and shorthand used by the writer.

Although Table 13.4 outlines a range of common data presentation forms, for many people reading research reports, tables, charts and diagrams are only seen through peripheral vision. They are rarely studied and can become like holes in the page; they don't really exist. This is because we do not teach people how to read tables and diagrams. The next section is an attempt to overcome this with the help of some guidelines.

How to read tables?

Firstly, we can define the purpose of a table as a way of producing a numeric photograph of a situation in long shot. Diamond and Jefferies (2001) suggest

Table 13.5 Example of a frequency table: age distribution of sample

Age group	No	(%)
<18	23	10.3
18–21	47	21.2
22–26	53	23.9
27–30	42	18.9
31–34	35	15.8
35+	22	9.9
Total	222	100.0

Table 13.6 Example of a cross-tabulation: parity of study sample by age group

	Primagravida		Multigravida	
Age group	No	(%)	No	(%)
<18	32	(17.5)	2	(1.0)
18–21	40	(21.9)	31	(15.3)
22–26	42	(23.0)	47	(23.1)
27–30	34	(18.5)	54	(26.6)
31–34	23	(12.6)	40	(19.7)
35+	12	(6.5)	29	(14.3)
Total	183	(100.0)	203	(100.0)

the aim of drawing a table is to transform a set of numbers into a format that is easy to understand. Although we are unlikely to admire it as much as a photograph, it does allow us to grasp the total picture, and then start to examine some of the individual details by zooming in to specific parts of the picture. This means we can answer specific questions we might have about it, such as 'do midwives see promoting sexual health as important as promoting effective parenting skills (Bennett et al 2001)?'

There are two different kinds of table; a *frequency table* and a *cross-tabulation* or *contingency table*. A frequency table looks at how often (frequently) categories of one variable occurred in the data. For example, Table 13.5 above illustrates a frequency table for age.

The second type of table takes the simple frequency table, and attempts to look for a pattern by introducing another variable, such as parity, so that the first variable is broken down into another variable. This is called a *cross-tabulation* or *contingency table*, where one factor is 'contingent' that is conditional or dependent on another. An illustration of this type of table is shown in Table 13.6 where parity is cross-tabulated with age.

When reading a table, the first task is to examine the layout and headings. Start by establishing what the table represents: this should be clearly conveyed in the title. Look carefully to see if it relates to just one variable, which would indicate a frequency table, or if it cross-tabulates two or more variables. This will help you anticipate what kind of a pattern it may contain. Then look at the columns and rows. Each should be clearly labelled at the top of the columns, and to the left of the rows. This helps you to 'read' the table in terms of what the numbers represent.

A useful starting point for a summary table is to look down each column for the highest numbers, to get a feel for which item or category was the largest and how large it was. Ask yourself 'is that what could have been anticipated?' How close in value are the other items to the highest? Again, is that what could have been expected, or is this an unexpected, clinically relevant finding? You can also consider the reverse of this by identifying which categories have the smallest values. Could they have been anticipated or is that unusual? Look too at the relative size or pattern in the value of all the numbers. This will give you some idea of the rank order of the items in terms of which is the highest, the next highest, and so on. Some tables may present the rows in terms of rank order as part of the format. Do these numbers go down gradually in size, or are there some items with large values followed by a sudden drop down to the next values? This will tell you if there is some consistency in the distribution, or whether most responses fell into a small number of categories that were mentioned by, or typical of, most people in the study.

Where there are a number of columns in the table, it is useful to make comparisons across each item indicated by the row headings to see if the value of the number in each column is similar or different. If different, are the differences small or large? As you start to identify patterns amongst the results, ask yourself the following questions:

◆ What does this suggest to me?
◆ Is this what I would expect or not?
◆ So what?

This type of reflection and analysis will allow you to come to some opinions about the findings and how they relate to the terms of reference. What could be the 'story' or explanation behind the findings? Your answers can then be compared with the researcher's comments on each table. Examine the tables before you read the researcher's comments, so that you do not simply accept what they say unquestioningly.

These points are also useful if you need to construct tables. The first point is to establish if the information will be easier to communicate in the form of a summary table. If the answer is 'yes', then you will need to identify how much information you need to put in each table. Avoid overloading the reader with too much information. However, sometimes it is easier to compare two situations, such as caesarian section rate between primigravida and multigravida women by putting them in the same table so making comparisons more evident.

Tables from randomized control trials (RCTs)

Where the table represents the results from an RCT there are certain conventions the researcher should observe. These include which variables are

Table 13.7 Example from an RCT showing satisfaction with method of administration of pain relief (reproduced with permission from Moffat et al 2001)

	(A) Self administration $n = 30$	(B) Staff administration $n = 30$	A vs. B Chi-square test
Satisfaction with method of administration [of pain relief]	30 (100%)	20 (66.7%)	$\chi^2 = 9.72, P{<}0.01$

shown as columns or rows. According to Coombes (2001), cross-tabulations are one way of representing how categories of one variable (independent variable) are distributed across the categories of another variable (dependent variable). The purpose is to allow the researcher to see whether there are any patterns of association. The column headings are used to display the independent variable and the row headings indicate the dependent variable. This can be seen in Table 13.7 above, which shows the results of women randomly allocated to a self-medication group and a traditional staff administration of pain relief group and the influence this had on the dependent variable of women's satisfaction with the method of pain relief administration (Moffat et al 2001). This layout allows the reader to examine differences in the dependent variable across the different forms of the independent variable, which above is given as the form of drug administration.

To help you answer the question what does the table show, the researcher will indicate if they have used inferential statistics on the table, and what was found. This is indicated either underneath the table or as a column in the summary table, as above, where the researcher should indicate the statistical test used, the result and the 'P' value, which indicates whether the differences could have happened purely by chance.

In this table there is a clear difference in the dependent variable of satisfaction with the method of administration of pain relief, by the independent variable of the method of administration. The researchers have used the chi-square test, which has the symbol χ^2. This produced a value of 9.72, which can be converted to a 'P' value (probability level) of <0.01. This means that the likelihood of this difference between the two groups happening by chance rather than relating to the method of administration is less than one in a hundred. In other words, satisfaction with the method of administration favours the self-administration method. Box 12.1 in Chapter 12 outlines how to interpret 'P' values.

Making sense of bar charts and pie charts

Although tables provide an overall view of data, and allow us to zoom in on specific parts, we have to interpret and keep track of a lot of ideas in our head. This means we have to visualize differences in size between quantities using their numeric short hand. Bar charts, histograms and pie charts are different, as they provide instant visual comparisons. Parahoo (1997) suggests that diagrammatic presentation of data is designed to attract the reader's attention and give a sense of proportion.

However, we still have to know something of the conventions surrounding such displays, so that we can read them easily. *Bar charts* contain a series of rectangles or 'blocks' presented either vertically or horizontally, and represent the values or scores for a number of categories. They are an ideal way of highlighting comparisons. This can be between two or more variables where the height of the bars will draw attention to differences between them. Good bar charts are presented in size order from the largest down to the smallest. This helps to follow differences in size.

The bar chart below extends the use of bar charts by providing a comparison between categories over time. Here three different points of time are shown to illustrate the difference between staff administering paracetamol for perineal pain and women self-medicating (Moffat et al 2001). The differences in the number of tablets taken at 48 and 72 hours are strikingly visible as a result of this form of presentation.

Histograms are similar in appearance to bar charts, but each block touches those on either side as the data they represent are on a continuous scale ranging from zero upwards. In most bar charts, the order of the blocks does not matter, as they are separate (discrete) items and could be reordered without changing the meaning. In histograms, this would be impossible, as with height, weight or frequency the order of the blocks cannot be rearranged without destroying the natural sequence.

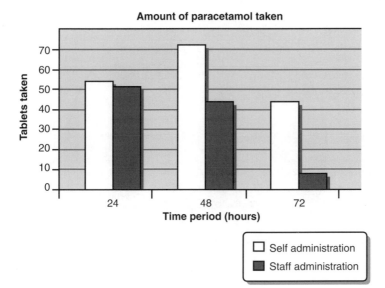

Fig. 13.2   Illustration of bar charts (reproduced with permission from Moffat et al 2001)

Making sense of bar charts, and histograms, is a matter of comparison between blocks and establishing the overall pattern on display. The important question to answer is 'how does this relate to the terms of reference (study aim)?' Is the pattern important to the research, and is it clinically important? In examining such charts a vital point is that the scale used by the author or publishers can make a small difference between two outcomes seem quite large, merely by making the scale of the diagram bigger. It is always wise, therefore, to look carefully at how big the differences are, and consider the question 'is the difference really remarkable, or does the scale of the figure exaggerate the relative differences?'

Pie charts are another form of what Martin and Thomson (2000) refer to as 'user friendly graphical presentations'. A pie chart is a circle 'sliced-up' to represent the relative proportion of each of the categories in a response. Their clarity can be seen from the example taken from Birch's (2001) work on the causes of stress in midwifery.

Here, not only can comparisons be made between the different variables, but the relationship of each variable to the bigger picture can be seen at a glance. So, stress from personal life can be seen to be small in relation to workload, which is the largest single stressor.

Pie charts work well with nominal or categorical levels of measurement, where all the items make up 100% of the total. The number of slices should normally be between three and six, providing that the sections are not too small to make comparisons difficult. Although Coombes (2001) describes how pie charts can be constructed with a protractor working on a basis of

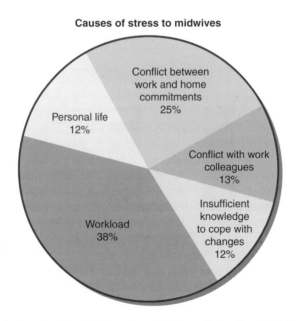

Causes of stress to midwives

Conflict between work and home commitments 25%

Personal life 12%

Conflict with work colleagues 13%

Insufficient knowledge to cope with changes 12%

Workload 38%

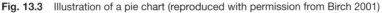

Fig. 13.3   Illustration of a pie chart (reproduced with permission from Birch 2001)

360°, nowadays they can be produced in minutes by means of a computer spreadsheet and chart-making program.

All the data presentation methods described in this section serve the same purpose, that is to convey the results of data analysis clearly, and meaningfully. The problem for the researcher is to show the results in a way that will best be assimilated by the reader, and will make the point. When it comes to the researcher choosing between a table and bar chart, Donnan (2000) suggests that tables are good at emphasizing particular numeric values and other forms such as bar charts and pie charts, show overall patterns. When reading research reports, all forms of presenting the data should be carefully examined; remember 'every picture tells a story'.

Inferential statistics

So far we have considered descriptive statistics in depth, and mentioned inferential statistics in passing. This last category is more complex than the previous one, and so in keeping with the aim of this book, which is to act as an introduction to key ideas in research, this section will be somewhat restricted, and simplified. Further, more in-depth details can be gained from some of the statistical texts already mentioned, as well as Hicks (1996), who provides a comprehensive source of support.

LoBiondo-Wood and Haber (2002) suggest that inferential statistics have two purposes, firstly to estimate the probability that characteristics found in a sample accurately reflect those that may exist in the population as a whole, and secondly, to test hypotheses about a population by manipulating elements within a sample.

The first aim is to allow the researcher to be reasonably confident that what was found in a sample is likely to be found in the population from which they were taken. We can relate this forwards to the next chapter on sampling methods to appreciate one of the basic assumptions of inferential statistics, and that is that the sample has been drawn using probability sampling methods. This means the sample was chosen in such a way as to ensure it is reasonably representative of the larger group. If this has been achieved, what we find in the sample should be found in a similar way in the larger group. The second aim, highlighted by LoBiondo-Wood and Haber (2002), relates to experimental designs where the researcher needs to identify whether any differences between the experimental and control groups are more likely to be due to the intervention variable, than the result of chance or some other explanation.

The major distinction in inferential statistics is between *parametric* and *non-parametric tests*. Parametric tests provide reasonably accurate answers to questions regarding the existence of real differences between groups or the likelihood of features of the sample being found in the wider population. However, they require a number of strict conditions to be met before they can be used. These include the following:

◆ The level of measurement for the variable must be interval or ratio (this is why understanding the levels of measurement is important).

- The distribution (spread) of the variable must be normally distributed (spread evenly either side of the mean to form a bell shaped curve if plotted on a graph).
- The spread of the measurements should be uniformly close to the mean and not include a large number of 'outliers'. This condition is referred to as 'homogeneity of variance'.

Despite these guidelines on the criteria for parametric tests you will find some rules being broken as it is argued that parametric tests are very robust and can cope with a certain amount of rule bending (Martin and Thomson 2001). The usual advice for the novice, however, is that where there is any doubt about the features of the data, use non-parametric tests. For each parametric test there is a non-parametric equivalent so that the same calculation can be made; however, the strength of the relationship indicated by the test may differ.

There are two main categories of inferential statistics commonly encountered in research reports; the first is those which seek to establish a consistent pattern or *correlation* between two variables, and the other is *tests of significance* which are used to establish cause and effect relationships, where tests of significance are used to establish if difference between groups could have happened merely by chance.

Correlation

This statistical calculation explores the relationship between two variables collected from each person or item in a sample (e.g. width of pelvis and length of labour), and attempts to assess if they are related. It is important to stress it does not attempt to say that one causes the other, only that some kind of pattern or association exists between them. Correlation is an attempt to answer the question 'to what extent are two variables related to each other in terms of *strength* – how closely are they related, and *direction* – are they positively related, that is, do measurements of both variables go up together, or down together, or are they negatively related, that is as one variable goes up the other goes down.

The strength of the relationship in correlation is measured by a *correlation coefficient*. This is a single number that is the product of a calculation that provides a measure of how closely the two variables are related. The correlation coefficient is measured on a scale between $+1$, which is a perfect positive correlation, and -1, a perfect negative correlation. When the calculation reveals that there is no relationship between two variables, the coefficient (the number that indicates the strength of the relationship) will be zero. In other words we are dealing with a scale that looks something like Figure 13.4.

An illustration will clarify the way in which all correlations lie somewhere on the line above. A perfect positive correlation between personal income and an individual's expenditure on clothes would mean that a 10% increase in income would result in an extra 10% increase in the amount spent on clothes. In the case of a negative correlation, it would mean that as measurements of one variable go up, for instance cost of travelling by train per

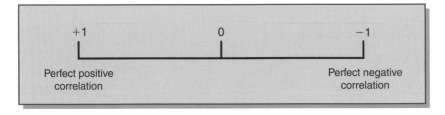

Fig. 13.4 Scale used to indicate correlation coefficient

kilometre, there would be a corresponding decrease in the number of rail passengers. A perfect negative correlation of −1 would be indicated when a 14% increase in the cost of rail fares per kilometre, would result in a 14% drop in the number of passengers.

The important point about correlation is that it measures *similarities*, whereas tests of significance, which are used in RCTs, measure *differences*. This is a key principle in understanding the different purposes of these two statistical techniques.

The usefulness of knowing a correlation exists, is that it allows us to plan, or make broad predictions that will be reasonably accurate, depending on the strength of the correlation. So for instance, we know that there is a reasonably strong positive relationship between social class and the number of mothers who breastfeed. This means that if geographical areas are compared using a scale of social class, it can be expected that the demand for support for breastfeeding will be higher in those areas with a higher social class distribution.

As there is rarely a perfect correlation between variables, a strong relationship will be anything from 0.05 up to 0.08. A medium relationship will be around 0.03 to 0.04. A strong negative relationship where the value of one variable goes up whilst another measure goes down, would be from −0.05 to −0.08. This means there is a consistent pattern, where one variable goes up the other goes down, e.g. as the numbers of staff receiving higher levels of continuing education go up, the numbers of complaints and litigation go down. A useful checklist of correlation levels and their meaning is shown in Table 13.8.

Calculating correlation

There are two main methods of calculating correlation, depending on the type of data being examined. Where one of the variables is measured using an ordinal level of measurement, such as a Likert scale, or other scale, such as Apgar score, where the precise difference between measures is not known, then Spearman's rho (pronounced 'row') is used. This is indicated by the symbol r_s. If the measurements for both variables in a correlation are at interval or ratio level, and if they comply to a number of other stringent criteria (see Clegg 1988 or Bowers 1997), then a more accurate method called

Table 13.8 Interpreting correlation

Where the correlation coefficient is:	
0.9 to +1	A very strong to perfect positive correlation
0.5 up to 0.8	A good to strong positive relationship
0.3 or 0.4	A reasonable positive relationship
0 to 0.2	No to little evidence of a positive relationship
0 to −0.2	No to little evidence of a negative or inverse relationship
−0.3 or −0.4	A reasonable negative or inverse relationship
−0.5 to −0.8	A good to strong negative or inverse relationship
−0.9 to −1	A very strong to perfect negative or inverse correlation

the Pearson product moment, usually referred to as Pearson r (or sometimes more informally as Pearson's r), is used.

Both measures use the same scale of between +1 and −1 to show the strength of the relationship between the two sets of measurements. Although Pearson r is a more accurate measurement, the nature of the measurements used in midwifery means that Spearman's rho is probably more commonly encountered.

More detail on calculating correlation can be found in books such as Clegg (1988) and Bowers (1997). Some authors such as Bowers (1997) and Salkind (2000) outline how to use computer programs such as SPSS (Statistical Package for the Social Sciences) and Minitab (another statistical computer package) to carry out these calculations. If you are carrying out correlation yourself these provide a good source of further information.

Multiple regression

Before leaving correlation, it is worth mentioning a natural development of the technique, which is multiple regression. Whereas correlation works on the relationship between two variables, multiple regression takes the same idea, but extends it to take into account a wider range of interval or ratio variables that might be related to a particular outcome at the same time. LoBiondo-Wood and Haber (2002) give the example of trying to establish which factors influence the decision to breastfeed. This is likely to be the result of a number of factors such as age, previous experience with breastfeeding, number of other children, and knowledge of the advantages of breastfeeding; all will play a part in shaping the decision to breastfeed.

Tests of significance

Tests of significance are crucial in clinical trials where the researcher attempts to demonstrate that the intervention they introduced had an effect on a dependent variable (outcome). They provide the researcher with the ability to rule out the element of chance by testing for significant differences between or among groups (Burns and Grove 2001).

In choosing a test of significance the researcher must ensure that the requirements for the application of the test are met by the data collected. Tests of significance can be either parametric or non-parametric. As indicated earlier, parametric tests provide the greatest degree of accuracy. A favourable statistical result using a parametric test is accepted as indicative of an important finding. However, the stringent conditions relating to the level of measurement and distribution of the data within the sample must be fulfilled before they can be used.

The conditions for using non-parametric tests are a lot easier to meet, and they can be used with much smaller data-sets compared to parametric tests, but the degree of accuracy is less. In other words the chances of being wrong in saying that real differences have been found between the groups in a study are greater when using a non-parametric test than when using a parametric equivalent. The difference between the data that can be used is again related to the level of measurement and also to whether the distribution of the variable meets the criteria of a normal distribution.

Some of the commonly encountered tests of significance are outlined in Table 13.9. Further details of these can be found in many of the texts mentioned in this chapter.

Conducting research

Although McMillan and Roberts (2001) admit that 'fledgling' health care researchers can feel intimidated by the prospect of using statistics in their studies, their importance to credible and successful findings means they cannot be ignored. The answer is to prepare yourself fully for this aspect of the research process, and seek help and support once you have decided to conduct quantitative research.

Remember that data analysis, according to Burns and Grove (2001), is probably the most exciting part of research, as it provides the answers to the questions that inspired the study. However, the analysis of data is not something the researcher thinks about only once data gathering is complete; the method of analysis has to be considered at the design stage. As each item in the tool of data collection is decided for inclusion in the study, the researcher should consider the level of measurement that will be required. The basic principle is to collect data at the highest level practical, so individual age should be sought rather than grouped data (ordinal) or even nominal level e.g. <21 or 21+, unless it is known for sure that calculations such as mean, median or standard deviation will not be crucial. Collecting data at the highest level ensures a greater choice in data presentation and analysis.

Use other researchers' findings to decide how you might present information, such as in the form of a table or other visual display. Will some variables need to be cross-tabulated with other items of information? I have often constructed 'dummy' tables at this point to explore the different ways data may be displayed. Decide which variables will be shown as columns and which in rows as well as the direction in which percentages will be calculated (row

Table 13.9 Common statistical tests and procedures you will encounter

Name of test	Type	Description
t-test Independent t-test Dependent t-test	Parametric test used on interval and ratio data	The independent t-test is used to compare the means of two separate groups. The dependent t-test measures two means in the same group, using a 'before and after/pre-test post-test' design.
Mann–Whitney U test	Non-parametric equivalent of the t-test.	Used to compare the means of two groups with ordinal data, where data are not normally distributed.
Wilcoxon test	The non-parametric equivalent of the dependent t-test	Used where scores are in pairs, such as pre-test post-test design, but where data are not normally distributed.
Chi-squared test (χ^2)	Non-parametric test The simple χ^2 uses nominal data, the complex χ^2 is used where there are three or more sets of data	Looks at whether the difference between two groups was as expected. Are the groups the same or different? Applies to nominal or ordinal data.
Pearson coefficient (Pearson r)	Parametric test that establishes the relationship between two interval or ratio variables	The size of the relationship is indicated on a scale between +1 and −1. Strong relationships are usually around 0.5 to 0.8 positive or negative.
Spearman's coefficient Spearman's rho ('row') r	This is the non-parametric version of the above and is used with nominal or ordinal data.	As above.

percentages or column percentages?). The appropriate statistical calculations or tests can also be written alongside the dummy tables.

The level of measurement will influence the options available for presentation, especially where graphical presentations are concerned. So, for instance, nominal and ordinal level data can be shown as a table, but are often clearer as a bar chart or pie chart. Interval and ratio level data can be displayed as a histogram not a bar chart, as they are suitable for continuous data. With a histogram the sides of adjacent blocks touch, unlike those of bar charts. Line graphs can also be used for interval and ratio data.

At the data input stage, the data from the raw questionnaires, observation checklists etc. will be entered on the computer. It is essential that any problem areas are anticipated and principles drawn up to solve dilemmas in data entry. Burns and Grove (2001) give some illustrations of this in regard to questionnaires. An example is where the respondent when faced with an instruction 'indicate which is the most important of the following' has indicated two items instead of one, or on a Likert scale has marked the space between two categories instead of indicating the specific point on the scale. The options are to omit that respondent from the analysis, or to take the first or highest/lowest in the options indicated.

Where a questionnaire contains open comments that are going to be turned into frequency counts in a table, a coding frame of categories has first to be constructed. The category 'other' can be reserved for the small number of responses that do not seem to fit any of the existing codes. Care has to be taken that the category 'other' does not become bigger than any of the other major groups developed; if it does, some sub grouping has to take place.

Quality control of data inputting should be initiated, especially where more than one person is involved in entering the data. The random checking of data entry sheets is worthwhile to confirm accuracy. Where the researcher is the only one inputting data, Burns and Grove (2001) suggest that sessions should not last more than two hours and attempts made not to break the rhythm of entry. They maintain that more mistakes are likely as time extends over the two-hour mark.

One of the first tasks of the data analysis stage is to summarize the data ready for statistical processing. Summarizing can be as simple as counting how many times options were chosen or occurred in a frequency distribution. This is carried out on the characteristics of the sample, such as age, parity, grade of staff, or whatever sample characteristics have been collected. At the planning stage the grouping or banding of some data might need to take place, so for instance lengths of time or age may be grouped (remembering the points made earlier on levels of measurement). The size of the bandings can be determined from previous research, but it is worth noting that too small a banding can lead to information overload and hide broader patterns; too large a banding will lose the sensitivity of some data in highlighting differences amongst smaller groupings.

One major error to avoid in grouping categories is overlapping the groups. Taking the example of age, there is no point in having one group 20 to 25 and then the next group 25 to 30, as 25 appears twice. It should be 20 to 25 then 26 to 30 and so on.

Once the data have been processed they can be selectively turned into visual displays. Most computers are now capable of producing tables and through spreadsheet programmes such as Excel© can present their content in a number of appropriate forms such as bar charts and pie charts. Interestingly, Martin and Thomson (2000) suggest avoiding the use of three-dimensional graphics as these detract from a presentation and are generally not well received by peer-reviewed journals and reviewers.

As with other aspects of the research process, it is important to pay attention to detail. Look at this aspect of the research as a crucial part of getting your points across. Unless the statistical elements in your research have been carried out professionally, and to a high standard, the credibility of your results will suffer.

Critiquing research

The purpose of this section has been to make you more familiar with some of the basic ideas related to statistical displays. These are most commonly encountered in the results sections of research papers or presentations. The immediate reaction of many people confronted by statistics is to panic. This is an emotional response that can be controlled. The information above has hopefully helped you to realize there is a logic and order to statistics that can be appreciated and understood.

When faced with a quantitative researcher paper, the first thing to do is to look very carefully at the labels attached to the tables and figures. What do they show? Then look at how this information is presented to you, and begin to read the story it reveals.

Look at tables or figures and ask yourself 'are these descriptive or inferential statistics?' If they are descriptive, you will need to examine the size of categories. How big was the study, what is the pattern of frequencies across the categories, which are the large frequencies, which are the small? Would I have anticipated the size of these? Look at the relative size between the categories; is there a slow step down in size or are there one or two large categories, and then a big drop in size before the next categories?

Whether it is a table or chart, can you read the story of what is going on? What does it say to you? Are there questions raised in your mind as a result of the pattern you see?

Where inferential statistics are used, look in or below the table, where there should be additional information such as the tests that have been carried out and the 'P' values that have been produced. This may even be in the methods sections under 'statistical analysis', or where the results are described. What does the size of these values suggest to you? The closer the 'P' value is to 1, the more likely the null-hypothesis is to be correct; the closer it is to zero (starting from a value of $P < 0.05$ going smaller) the more likely the alternative hypothesis of a real difference between the groups is to be true.

In the case of an RCT, has the author demonstrated that the groups were comparable to start with? If not, is there anything about the differences that could play a part in interpreting the results? Similarly, in the case of an RCT, could the numbers dropping out of any of the groups have made a difference to the meaningful comparisons between the groups?

Once you have searched the figures and tables for meaning, read through the text to see what the writer makes of all this. Do they talk you through the tables and point out things that you may not have noticed, or explained what the results meant for them? Where the data raised questions in your mind, do the authors answer those questions for you?

Where there are unfamiliar statistical elements or things you have forgotten, check them out in a good statistics reference book. Depending on where the article is published, you may feel questions such as whether the authors have used appropriate statistical procedures or tests should have been established by the journal. Be aware that you will not be able to make that assumption with all journals.

Do not ignore tables and figures. Do try and get something out of them. Each time you do this thorough analysis, you will learn a little bit more, and become more relaxed about reading the statistical elements in a study.

Key Points

◆ Collecting quantitative data means that statistical processes will be involved in the analysis stage. Understanding the principles behind these processes is important in correctly interpreting the findings of research.

◆ Research findings are presented following certain conventions and use presentation methods such as tables, bar charts, histograms and pie charts. Every picture tells a story; so these should never be overlooked.

◆ Statistics fall into two main categories of descriptive and inferential statistics. Users of research need to know the principles and assumptions on which these are based, as well as those relating to parametric and non-parametric tests.

◆ The level of measurement of the data will influence many of the decisions made in the research process. An understanding of these levels is crucial to understanding why certain decisions are made in the choice of statistical techniques.

◆ Although the jargon and symbols used in statistics may look intimidating, in reality a basic understanding is not difficult to achieve. Competency in understanding basic statistical principles to research data is essential to applying research to practice.

References

Bennett N, Blundell J, Malpass L and Lavender T (2001) Midwives' views on redefining midwifery 2: public health. British Journal of Midwifery 9(12): 743–746.

Birch L (2001) Stress in midwifery practice: an empirical study. British Journal of Midwifery 9(12): 730–734.

Bowers D (1996) Statistics From Scratch For Health Care Professionals. Chichester: John Wiley.

Bowers D (1997) Further Statistics From Scratch For Health Care Professionals. Chichester: John Wiley.

Burns N and Grove S (2001) The Practice of Nursing Research: Conduct Critique and Utilization (4th edn). Philadelphia: W.B. Saunders.

Carter J, Johanson R, Heycock E, Sultan A, Walklate K and Jones P (2001) Long-term health after childbirth. British Journal of Midwifery 9(12): 748–753.

Clegg F (1982) Simple Statistics. Cambridge: Cambridge University Press.

Cluett E (2000) An introduction to statistics in midwifery research. In: Cluett E and Bluff R (eds) Principles and Practice of Research in Midwifery. Edinburgh: Baillière Tindall.

Coombes H (2001) Research Using IT. Houndmills: Palgrave.

Crichton N (2001) Principles of statistical analysis in nursing and healthcare research. Nurse Researcher 9(1): 4–25.

Diamond I and Jefferies J (2001) Beginning Statistics: An Introduction for Social Scientists.

Donnan P (2000) Quantitative analysis (descriptive). In: Cormack D (ed.) The Research Process in Nursing (4th edn). Oxford: Blackwell.

Hicks C (1996) Undertaking Midwifery Research: A Basic Guide to Design and Analysis. New York: Churchill Livingstone.

Lavender T, Moffat H and Rixon S (2000) Do we provide information to women in the best way? British Journal of Midwifery 8(12): 769–775.

Lavender T, Bennett N, Blundell J and Malpass L (2001) Midwives' views on redefining midwifery 1: health promotion. British Journal of Midwifery 9(11): 666–670.

LoBiondo-Wood G and Haber J (2002) Nursing Research: Methods, Critical Appraisal, and Utilization (5th edn). St.Louis: Mosby.

Parahoo K (1997) Nursing Research: Principles, Process and Issues. Houndmills: Macmillan

Martin C and Thomson D (2000) Design and Analysis of Clinical Nursing Research Studies. London: Routledge.

McMillan I and Roberts P (2001) Editorial. Nurse Researcher 9(1): 3.

Moffat H, Lavender T and Walkinshaw S (2001) Comparing administration of paracetamol for perineal pain. British Journal of Midiwifery 9(11): 690–694.

Salkind N (2000) Statistics For People Who (Think They) Hate Statistics. Thousand Oaks: Sage.

Steen M and Marchant P (2001) Alleviating Perineal Trauma. RCM Midwives Journal 4(8): 256–259.

CHAPTER FOURTEEN

Sampling Methods

The outcome of any research project is dependent on both the reliability of the method used, and the type and quality of the sample on which the results are based. In this chapter the issues relating to who or what is included in the sample, and the alternative methods for choosing the sample, known as *sampling strategies*, will be examined.

First we must clarify the difference between a *'population'* and *'sample'*. Although these terms appear to be used almost interchangeably, there is a clear difference between them. The population is the total group of people, things or events the researcher is interested in saying something about, e.g. midwives who have a higher degree, women who have a home delivery, etc. Sampling is a process of selecting individuals who are representative of the population being studied (Burns and Grove 2001).

There are a number of alternative ways of arriving at a sample. The choice will vary depending on whether the research approach can be described as:

◆ Experimental
◆ Survey
◆ Qualitative.

The method of choosing the sample will also be influenced by how far the researcher wants to generalize the findings to the wider population. The more important it is to achieve this, the more complex the sampling strategy used.

Whatever the purpose of the study, the researcher is faced with three vital questions:

◆ Who or what will make up the sample?
◆ How are they to be chosen?
◆ How many will be chosen?

The chapter will illustrate the way in which the researcher attempts to answer these questions.

Why sample?

Why bother to sample in the first place? Surely it must be more accurate to get information from a total group? In terms of practicalities, it will not always be possible to collect information from an entire group. For example, we cannot send a questionnaire to every pregnant woman in Britain, as many would have delivered before we found out who should be included. It can also be extremely expensive to gather information from a total group, and it may not always be that much more accurate than a sample anyway.

LoBiondo-Wood and Haber (2002) believe that providing an appropriate sampling strategy has been used it is almost always possible to obtain a reasonably accurate understanding of a phenomenon under investigation by obtaining data from a sample.

The aim of sampling is to select a sample in such a way that it has the minimum of bias, and represents the characteristics of those in the population as closely as possible. A biased sample would consist of people, events or things, which were very different from those in the total group. An example of a biased sample would be a study which used a group of pregnant midwives to 'stand for' pregnant women in general and ask how they intended feeding their baby. We would expect there to be a difference between this sample and the total population of pregnant women, that would make decisions made on the results unreliable.

It is clear from this that the method of sampling deserves a great deal of attention. We should ensure that it has been planned in such a way as to recognize and minimize potential bias.

Inclusion/exclusion criteria

Before we select our sample we need to define our population accurately. This is achieved by specifying *inclusion* and *exclusion criteria*. Inclusion criteria are the characteristics we want those in our sample to possess. This is why it is sometimes referred to as *eligibility criteria*. Examples of inclusion criteria would be women who have a normal vaginal delivery at term, or women in certain age groups with no complications of pregnancy. In other words, it is the characteristics they must possess to allow them to stand for the general group we want to say something about.

Exclusion criteria consist of those characteristics we do not want those in our sample to have because it may make them untypical and so bias the results. There may be other reasons for excluding some people from a study, such as the risk of harm for those with a certain condition or characteristic.

The researcher must consider the inclusion and exclusion criteria at the planning stage. These should be clearly stated in any report for the reader to consider whether they could lead to some limitations in applying the results to other groups. Clear examples of inclusion and exclusion criteria are usually found in randomized control trials (RCTs) that are very sensitive to the element of bias. So for example, the following appears in the study by Moffat et al (2001) that compared patient- and midwife-administered oral analgesia in the postnatal period:

> *The eligibility criteria consisted of primigravida women who were admitted to a low-risk postnatal word following a normal vaginal delivery that had resulted in a first or second-degree tear (regardless of whether they were sutured). Exclusions were women requiring high dependency postnatal care and those who had experienced a multiple birth, episiotomy, third degree tear or post-partum haemorrhage.*
> (p. 690)

Sampling methods

At this point we must recognize that different research approaches will require different sampling methods, although some methods can be used in a variety of approaches. In any situation the researcher must try to draw the sample in such a way as to:

◆ Reduce sampling bias
◆ Increase representativeness.

Sampling bias, according to Polit et al (2001) is the systematic over-representation or under-representation of some segment of the population in terms of a characteristic relevant to the research question. Where bias is avoided, or minimized, there is a greater chance that the results can be applied to situations other than the one in which the data were gathered. In other words, it is easier to generalize from the results.

Bias can be reduced if the researcher can increase the representativeness of those chosen for the sample. They should be similar to the population they represent as closely as possible in ways that might influence the outcome of the study. This would include variables such as parity, social class, age and key attitudes and experiences. The researcher should establish the distribution of such variables in the population and then demonstrate statistically that the sample does not differ significantly from the total group in the possession of those characteristics.

What are the alternative sampling strategies available? Table 14.1 outlines the main methods available linked to the various broad research approaches.

Table 14.1 Sampling method by broad research approach

Research approach	Sampling method
Experimental	Cohort
	Simple random
	Stratified sampling
	Proportionate random
Quasi-experimental and ex post facto	Cohort
	Comparative groups
	Systematic random
Survey	Cohort
	Simple random
	Stratified random
	Proportionate random
	Systematic random
	Opportunity/convenience/accidental
	Quota
Qualitative	Purposive
	Convenience
	Snowball/network/chain/nominated
	Theoretical

Experimental sampling approaches

As we saw in Chapter 12, experiments have a particular function in research and that is to establish the presence of cause and effect relationships. In order to achieve this, sampling is carried out in very meticulous ways so that an accurate conclusion can be deduced from the findings. The method of sampling is drawn from a number of options grouped under the heading of *random sampling methods*. These options form what are called *probability sampling* methods. Using this approach, every unit in the population, whether it is people, things or events, should have an equal chance of being selected. If this criterion is achieved, it means that some of the sophisticated statistical tests can be used on the results. These allow the probable accuracy of statements made about the results to be calculated. Some of the alternative sampling methods in experimental design are:

◆ Cohort
◆ Simple random sample
◆ Stratified sample
◆ Proportional sampling.

Cohort

For a probability sample it is possible to use a total group rather than a proportion of them, providing this is practical and feasible. Examples would include all midwives working in one particular unit; all women discharged over the months of June and July; the last fifty people who attended a particular antenatal clinic, etc. If all of these people were included they would form a cohort, which means a total group within certain parameters such as diagnosis or time period. If each person (sampling unit) were included they would have a 100% chance of being selected, which fits the criteria of having an equal chance of being included in the study.

In an experimental design the cohort could act as their own control group and receive both an experimental intervention, followed by the control intervention, or vice versa. An alternative would be the random allocation of half the group to the experimental group, and half to the control group.

It is worth emphasizing that there are limitations to the use of cohorts. A total group in one situation may have a different mix of characteristics to a cohort in another area. This would make generalizations difficult. Similarly, it is assumed in using a cohort, that one group will be much like another. That is, those who form a group in one time period will be similar to those in another time period. This may not be the case as groups selected will differ over time as experiences, values as well as expectations can all change over time. Cohorts, then, have limitations in the extent to which they are similar to other cohorts and can be compared to those in different time periods.

Simple random sample

In many experimental situations it is not possible or desirable to take a total group as the sample, and a simple random sampling design is used instead.

12	57	42	14	01	84	35	21	75	33	61	68	32
85	83	35	22	13	38	47	90	15	65	74	40	09
10	39	55	86	16	03	91	75	62	34	11	59	17
22	08	60	13	26	99	71	40	91	69	35	04	65
49	74	26	39	09	16	87	56	20	54	88	93	82
36	06	33	47	98	49	07	19	51	27	43	71	54

Box 14.1 Example of a part of a table of random numbers

This is perhaps one of the most commonly misunderstood concepts in sampling. Many people assume that choosing a random sample is a haphazard, casual or indiscriminate way of selecting people for study. The word 'random' is assumed to imply that there is very little system applied to this process, which is far from the truth.

It is important to first of all differentiate between selecting a random sample and *random allocation*. In a random sample those eligible to be included in the study are identified from the larger population, and selected for inclusion in the research. This does not mean they have agreed to be included in the study, or that they will willingly take part. In the view of some researchers, findings can only be generalized if random sampling has taken place.

Random allocation, on the other hand, is frequently used in health service experimental research and is based on those who have agreed to take part in a study, and are willing to be allocated into either the experimental or control group. There is no guarantee that those who agree to take part in a random allocation research project are similar to the wider population. Random allocation is the system by which individuals are allocated to either the experimental or control group so that there is no element of bias surrounding who ends up in which group.

In order to achieve a random sample the researcher must have a complete list, or *sampling frame*, of all those who could be included in the sample. A sampling frame can be defined as a list of the total population who meet the inclusion and exclusion criteria of the study. Once the frame is constructed, each individual is consecutively given a number that can be used to identify them.

Individuals are then selected for inclusion in the study using a table of random numbers or list of computer-generated random numbers. Box 14.1 illustrates a small portion of a table of random numbers. These can be found in many research textbooks, books on statistics, and it is also possible to buy books of random number tables. In all such tables there is no systematic sequence to the way in which the numbers are listed. That is, they do not go up or down in any particular pattern, or are listed in an alternating odd/even way.

Using a table of random numbers

How do we randomly allocate people in an experiment? Let us imagine the researcher has gained the agreement of 50 women and has decided to allocate 25 to an experimental group, and 25 to the control group. A sampling frame of the names of the 50 women is first constructed. The order of the names is not important. Everyone is given a number in sequence from 1 to 50. Then 25 numbers between 1 and 50 are extracted from the table of random numbers to form the experimental group. The remaining 25 women whose number has not been picked will form the control group.

The method of selecting the numbers can now be described. Without looking closely at the table of random numbers, the researcher puts a finger down on to the page and looks for the number closest to it. For the purpose of illustration let us say the number 83 has been identified. This is the second number in the second column in Box 14.1. As this is above 50, which is the number of people who have been allocated a number, it is ignored. Keeping the finger on the page, the researcher now moves their finger, right, left, up or down, or diagonally in any direction. As they move their finger each number between 1 and 50 is accepted, and any above 50 rejected. If a number has already been selected it is also rejected until 25 different numbers have been drawn. So let us assume, having started at 83, we continue to move in a straight line to the right along the row. This would give us numbers 35, 22, 13, 38, and 47. Number 90 would be rejected, and 15 accepted. At any point the researcher may alter direction, or lift their finger and replace it at a different point. It really does not matter.

Once the 25 numbers have been drawn, those people who have been allocated each of those numbers will be identified from the sampling frame. These will form the people in the experimental group. Anyone with a number not included in the 25 drawn at random would be in the control group.

How would this work in the case of an RCT where a sampling frame could not be constructed? For example, if people were to be selected for a prospective study as they entered the system, say at a booking clinic?

In this case the researcher would use sealed envelopes. The table of random numbers would be used in the same way as just described where if the researcher again wished to use two groups of 25 women, 25 numbers would be picked out, and designated the experimental group. A pack of envelopes would then be numbered from 1 to 50. In those envelopes whose number corresponded with one of the 25 numbers drawn from the random table, a slip of paper saying 'experimental group' or stating the experimental intervention would be placed in the envelope. All the other envelopes would have a slip indicating 'control group' or the control intervention, or no intervention where an experimental variable was being compared to no intervention.

The envelopes would then be placed in number sequence from 1 to 50. As each person who had agreed to take part entered the study, the researcher would open the next envelope in sequence, and follow the instructions.

In the example of a table of random numbers it should be clear that the table used would only be applicable if the total number of people in the sampling frame was under 100. This is because as the numbers are in pairs, the maximum number would be 99. For larger studies, it is possible to use tables or computer generated numbers with three digit numbers that would be applicable for sampling frames extending up to 999.

Stratified sample

The basic principle of a simple random sample is that everyone has an equal chance of being selected for either the experimental or control group. There are cases, however, where this method may result in an over-representation of certain characteristics in one of the groups. So, for instance, the experimental group could have mainly primagravid women and the control group mainly multigravid women.

To avoid this the researcher can first stratify the sample into parity, and then sample within each parity appropriately. In the case of a prospective experimental design the researcher would use numbered envelopes for each parity group. Once it is established whether the individual agreeing to take part in the study is primigravida or multigravida, the next envelope in the appropriate pile is opened. This way there should be an even spread of primigravid and multigravid women in both the experimental and control group.

Proportionate sampling

A further refinement of the stratified sample is the proportionate sample. Here, the number of participants should be selected in proportion to their occurrence in the population (Burns and Grove 2001). So with the example of parity, it could be felt important that the sample should reflect the proportion of primigravid to multigravid women within each experimental and control group. If there were a proportion of 60% multigravid women delivering in a particular unit to 40% primigravid, then a proportional sample would also provide a sample with the same ratio between parities.

Quasi-experimental and ex post facto designs

Chapter 12 discussed alternatives to RCTs such as quasi-experimental and ex post facto designs. Quasi-experimental designs are used where it is not possible, usually for reasons such as ethical difficulties or practical constraints, to randomly allocate people to experimental and control groups. In these circumstances groups already formed and in existence are used. Examples would be women on two different wards, or couples attending two different locations for antenatal classes. One location is used for the experimental group, and the other for the control group. This is very similar to using two different cohorts in order to make a comparison.

The difficulty of this design is that it is not possible to rule out bias due to the blend of characteristics in each group. In other words, there may be important differences within the groups that may influence the outcome following an experimental intervention. Although this is a fundamental sampling weakness, in many cases this choice of design is the only one available. In these circumstances the researcher will attempt to illustrate the comparability between the two groups by identifying and describing key demographic characteristics, such as age, parity, social class, etc.

As there is an unequal difference in the chance of people ending up in the experimental as opposed to the control group (everyone on one ward would have a 100% chance and those on the comparison or control ward would have 0% chance), this is known as a non-probability sampling method. This is not as accurate a means of detecting true differences between groups as a probability sampling method, and for this reason non-probability sampling methods are less respected than probability methods. A non-probability sampling method has the advantage, however, of being practical, and often the best that can be done under the circumstances.

Ex post facto studies, also discussed in Chapter 12, are very similar to the quasi-experimental approach in the sampling methods used. The term means 'after the fact' and relates to the formation of groups that have already taken place before the start of the study and differ in relation to the independent variable. The researcher does not introduce the variable, but looks for groups or individuals who share a common identity on the basis of their own past decision to adopt a characteristic, such as smoking or behaviour, such as deciding to breastfeed. Again this is a non-probability method and we cannot generalize the findings to other situations with the same confidence as we can with probability sampling methods.

Survey methods

Although experimental designs are important to changing the culture of maternity care (West et al 2001), a far more frequently used approach to research in midwifery is that of the survey. Here some of the sampling methods already mentioned can be used and fall into both the probability and non-probability sampling methods.

Cohort

Surveys can first of all be based on a total group or cohort where all those in one particular group are sent a questionnaire, interviewed or observed. Examples would be all those attending antenatal classes in one venue, or all women giving birth to twins over a 6-month period. In survey methods, the strength of using a cohort is that it reduces the element of sampling error. If only some from a group are included in a sample, they may not accurately represent the characteristics of the full group. Where everyone in the group is included this kind of error cannot exist.

The limitation of using cohorts in surveys is that total groups can be too large to include everyone. They also suffer from the assumption, identified under experiments that one group is much like another, and that may not be the case. Factors such as seasonal variations or social class may make one group very different from another.

Simple random sampling

Surveys are very powerful where they are based on a simple random sample. Here, everyone from the total population has an equal chance of being included in the survey. The method has been described above under experiments where a sampling frame containing everyone fitting the inclusion criteria is constructed; a table of random numbers is then used to pick out the appropriate number of individuals for inclusion in the survey.

The advantage of using this method is that it is possible to make generalizations concerning the wider population on the basis of a random sample. This is because it falls into the category of probability sampling methods. One disadvantage of this method, however, is the difficulty of constructing a suitable sampling frame where there are a large number of eligible individuals in the target population, or where no list of likely individuals exists.

Stratified sampling

The process of simple random sampling in surveys can be refined further by dividing those eligible to be included in the sample into appropriate strata and then sampling from within each of the groups created. Examples of this would include grouping women by parity, or in the case of midwives, grade, or length of service.

The advantage of a stratified sample is that it ensures that those from relevant subgroups are included in the study. The disadvantages include the difficulty of predicting which subgroups might make a difference to the outcome, and then the problem of dividing the sampling frame into those characteristics. For instance, if it was thought that women with high self-esteem were more likely to breastfeed in relation to those with medium or low self-esteem, it would be difficult to first divide the target group into strata by level of self-confidence without the prior use of a scale measuring self-esteem.

Proportionate sampling

Proportionate sampling in a survey would be an attempt to achieve subgroups within the sample that were similar in proportion to the broader population. The aim of this would be to ensure that an unrepresentative proportion in one group did not produce a biased result. An example would be a survey of midwives' views on a particular aspect of midwifery. To ensure that the influence of grade was kept constant the population would first be stratified according to grade, then the numbers selected from each group would mirror the proportion in each grade in the total population. Again, this example would use a sampling frame and table of random numbers, or computer generated random numbers.

The advantage of this approach is a greater chance of accuracy and reduction in bias. The problems are similar to stratified sampling, and that is the difficulty of having prior knowledge of the size and location of some of the subgroups.

Systematic sampling

In some surveys where individuals, or objects, are being selected for inclusion from a very large population, systematic sampling is used in order to gain elements across the entire population. This is achieved by numbering all those who fit the inclusion criteria, then using a table of random numbers. The first number is selected randomly, and then individuals are selected following a predetermined frequency, such as every 5th, 10th or with very long lists every 20th, 50th or even 100th person or object.

The sampling interval, that is the distance between each unit in the sample, can be determined by first deciding on the total number required in the sample and then dividing that into the total number in the group. An example would be a questionnaire to a sample of women who had delivered in a particular unit over a 3-year period. If it was decided that the sample size required should be 80, and there were 3472 deliveries, then dividing that number by 80 would give a sampling interval of every 43rd person.

In order to ensure that women from the whole of the 3 years were represented, all those discharged could be numbered, using a table of random numbers the first number could be drawn out, for example 33, and then every 43rd number following that in the sampling frame would be chosen. So number 33 would be included, then 76, 119, 162 and so on. This would provide an even spread across the 3 years. Because the first number had been chosen randomly, it would conform to the criteria of a probability sample.

Cluster sampling

Where the elements in the sampling frame are geographically spread, or where the individual elements making up a population are unknown, a multi-stage approach called cluster sampling can be used (Burns and Grove 2001).

Imagine a national survey of the opinions of GPs regarding how they perceived the role of the midwife in providing care for women in the community. A sampling frame of all GPs would be a tall order; instead, the researchers may first produce a sampling frame of all health regions within Britain, and randomly select say a sample of ten regions. For each region they could then construct a sampling frame of districts. From this a total of three districts from each area may be chosen. The final sampling frame may be a list of all GP practices within the districts randomly chosen. From this a total of 20 GP practices could be randomly chosen and all the GPs in those practices sent questionnaires.

It is clear from this example why it is called *multi-stage sampling*. At each stage a sampling frame is constructed, and a simple random sample selected. Each level consists of the construction of the next sampling frame until the size of the units is manageable. The advantage of this system is that it can achieve an accessible sample from an almost impossible total population. The disadvantage is that the number of layers to the sampling process increases the degree of sampling error (Polit et al 2001). In other words, there will be a margin of error in the extent to which those left in the sample mirror the characteristics of those in the total population. Despite this drawback, its practical approach makes it a popular method in large-scale studies that have a problem in drawing an accessible sample.

Convenience/opportunity/accidental sampling

These three terms are often used to describe the same approach to sampling where the researcher includes in the study those people to whom they have easy access, and who happen to be in the right place at the right time. Hicks (1996) also uses the term incidental sample to describe the same situation where the researcher selects the most easily accessible people from the population. This is the method used by market researchers where people are stopped in the street and asked to answer questions. It is this method that people frequently mistake for a random sample.

This, and the next two methods described below, fall into the category of non-probability sampling methods, as everyone does not have the same chance of being included in the study. There is then no way of knowing whether those in these types of sample are representative or not. The ability to generalize from the findings is therefore restricted. Nevertheless, these approaches continue to be very popular because they are very practical in gaining quick and easy access to a sample, and provide an indication of possible responses to questions.

Examples of convenience samples might be women attending a particular antenatal clinic on a certain day, or midwives attending a study day who might be asked their opinions on some midwifery issue. The relevance of terms such as convenience or opportunity can be clearly seen from these examples.

The advantage of this approach is that it is simple. It is also cheap, quick and does not require the construction of elaborate sampling frames. The disadvantage is that of sampling bias, in that those who happen to be around a particular location may not be typical of the wider population they are taken to represent. Polit et al (2001) also warn that non-probability samples are rarely representative of the target population, as some segments of the population are likely to be systematically under-represented. An important point, however, is the extent to which there is variation in the population of the variable being studied, where the variation in a certain variable in the population is not that great, the risk of bias may be low, but where it is a very mixed or heterogeneous population the risk of bias is greater.

Quota sampling

This method is a refinement of convenience sampling as it attempts to produce a sample that is similar in certain key characteristics to the total population. The market researcher will use quota sampling by selecting so many people in certain age groups or occupation groups in order to argue that the sample is 'similar in structure' to the total population. In midwifery, there may be a similar attempt to include quotas such as so many women who are primigravida and so many multigravida, or in various age groups, or have experienced certain types of labour.

In many respects quota sampling is similar in purpose to stratified sampling, but it differs from a stratified sample in that the participants are not randomly selected from each strata.

The advantage of quota sampling is that the researcher is in a stronger position to say that because the sample is similar to the total population, then the results may be reasonably representative. The disadvantages are similar to stratified sampling, in that there is an assumption that the sub-groupings that may make a difference to the results are already known, and that the size of each of the groups is also known so that quotas can be calculated. It also depends on the information that allocates respondents to either one quota or another being easily ascertained from potential respondents.

Purposive sampling

This alternative, also known as *judgemental sampling* involves the researcher handpicking those in the sample on the basis of the researcher's knowledge of characteristics they know the individual possesses. Although this seems like producing a biased sample, its aim is to achieve the opposite, by ensuring that a range of opinions or experiences is included.

The advantages of this method are that the sample is known to possess key characteristics felt should be included in the survey. It is very practical, and efficient of time and money. The disadvantages highlighted by LoBiondo-Wood and Haber (2002) include the assumption that errors of judgement in over-representing or under-representing elements of the population in the sample will tend to balance out. This can be by no means clearly established. They also suggest that the more heterogeneous the population the more chance there is of introducing bias. Finally, they suggest that a constant problem with this method is that of conscious bias in the selection of individuals. This makes generalizations from the results very difficult.

Surveys, then, can be based on a variety of sampling methods. Some of these will result in statistical precision where probability sampling methods have been used. Where these are employed, reasonably large samples may be sought, and chosen from the wider population using random sampling approaches based on accurate sampling frames. The aim of this kind of survey is to be able to generalize the results to the wider population. Other approaches based on non-probability sampling methods are less precise, but a lot easier to conduct. Although it is difficult to judge their accuracy, they can provide useful 'snapshots' of situations that can be used as the basis for action.

Qualitative approaches

As qualitative research differs in so many respects from quantitative research, it is no surprise to find that the approach to sampling is also different. Because the aim is not to achieve a large representative sample from which generalizations can be made, sampling is not based on probability methods. The aim is rather to gather information from people who can provide inside information on specific kinds of experiences or who are part of a particular culture or subgroup different from the midwife. In terms of inclusion criteria, the most important factor is that they have knowledge or experience of the topic or phenomenon under examination. Those who are part of a qualitative study do not 'stand for' the larger population, in the same way as in quantitative research; they are included on the basis that they are members of an appropriate group. For this reason, as Holloway and Wheeler (1996) note, the rules of qualitative sampling are less rigid that those of quantitative methods, where a strict sampling frame is established before the research starts. The main alternatives include the following:

◆ Purposive
◆ Convenience
◆ Snowball/network/chain/nominated sample
◆ Theoretical.

Purposive sampling

We are already familiar with purposive sampling where the researcher includes individuals, or events on the basis of the researcher's knowledge of their relevance for the purpose of the study. Streubert and Carpenter (1999) point out that in qualitative studies there is no need to randomly select individuals because manipulation and control are not the purpose of the exercise.

According to Morse and Field (1996), the two principles that guide qualitative sampling are *appropriateness* and *adequacy*. They define appropriateness as participants who can best inform the research according to the requirements of the study. Adequacy is defined as the ability to develop full and rich descriptive data on the phenomenon in the study from the sample units.

Convenience sample

Just as the purposive sample provides the researcher with relevant information, so the convenience sample within qualitative research is relevant as long as those at hand have necessary information or experience relevant to the purpose of the study. The convenience sample can be used in both phenomenological studies and ethnographic research where the researcher draws on the experiences and activities of those who just happen to be in the setting being observed, or under study. The appropriateness of this method again illustrates the flexibility in this approach to data collection.

Snowball/network/chain/nominated sampling

All of these terms can be applied to the situation where the researcher may identify some individuals who possess the necessary characteristics or experiences, and then asks them to suggest others who may be willing to participate in the study. Holloway and Wheeler (1996) point out that this kind of sampling method is used where the researcher finds it difficult to identify useful informants, or where individuals cannot be easily contacted or where anonymity is desirable. In many of these cases sampling frames just do not exist.

Burns and Grove (2001) point out that the advantage of this method is that friends tend to have characteristics in common and therefore it is a good way to collect a sample of people who share the characteristic under study. They go on to warn that biases are built into this sampling procedure, as subjects are not independent of each other. This may not, however, be a problem.

Theoretical sampling

In qualitative research theoretical sampling is frequently used as a way of selecting the sample, and as a way of knowing when to stop data gathering. This is based on the principle that those in the sample can provide examples of the concepts or theoretical issues which are the concern of the research (Holloway and Wheeler 1996). This helps to determine who will be included in the sample. Data collection continues until no new insights are gained, and there is a repetition of information already gained. This is called theoretical saturation. At this point data collection is stopped.

Sampling in qualitative research is usually prospective and the researcher in ethnographic research will search out those in the setting it is believed will provide insights of use to the developing understanding of the topic.

Sample size

One of the most difficult tasks for the researcher is to establish at the planning stage how many people, things or events are going to be included in the sample. As the type of study to a large extent, influences the size of a sample, it is useful to consider the question of size under each of the headings already used in this chapter.

Experimental designs

As experimental designs are concerned with accuracy, there are some statistical guidelines the researcher can use in choosing a suitable sample size. The important factor is the size of the difference the researcher is looking for between the results of the experimental group and the control group before they are willing to say that an intervention has been successful. Unfortunately, for many conditions or situations, the difference between one group and another when measured on physiological outcomes may be quite small. This would mean that for differences to show up, the study would have to include quite a large number of people before that difference was clearly visible, and statistically relevant.

A statistical procedure called *power analysis* can be used to estimate the total size of the sample needed, given an anticipated difference in the results between two groups (LoBiondo-Wood and Haber 2002). However, in midwifery the number of experimental studies is relatively small, and some of those undertaken can be quite modest in sample size. It is often practical considerations such as time and resources that dictate the size of experimental groups. Closely examining the literature for the size of previous studies can be a great help to the researcher. It is also important to realize that it is not so much the total number of people to be admitted to a trial that is important, but the size of the subgroups used in the analysis of the results. Where the sample is divided into differences such as parity, or age, the size of the groups can be quite small, even though the overall group might have been quite large at the start.

One problem in experimental designs is the drop out rate from the study. This is referred to as *subject mortality* or *attrition*. Although the size of the sample can seem large to start, if the study is carried out over a long time period, or consists of several periods of testing and data collection, some people for one reason or another may be lost to the study. This can have consequences where there is a larger proportion dropping out of one of the groups as it can lead to an imbalance between the groups so that they may no longer be comparable. The best the researcher can do is to try and make the size of the groups as large as is practical, and to ensure that the size is reasonably in line with any previous research.

Surveys

The optimum sample size in surveys is variable, as it relates to the size of the total population. In surveys where the aim is to be able to generalize quite accurately to the total population, the sample size may be in the hundreds, but in other studies, where the total population itself is quite small, such as the number of male midwives, the sample may be quite small.

In choosing the sample size, the advice is to attempt to gain as large a sample as possible on the grounds that the larger the sample, the more representative it is likely to be (Polit et al 2001). However, there is also agreement that a large sample does not compensate for poor sampling methods. The important point made by Polit et al (2001) is that the ultimate criterion for assessing a sample is its representativeness. In other words, the researcher should be concerned with the quality of the sampling method and the extent to which it avoids bias, rather than simply including as large a number as possible.

As with experimental studies, it is often practical considerations that influence sample size. These include time, money and the availability of subjects. The researcher should also consider the extent to which the variables included in the survey vary in the population. The more something varies, the larger the sample needed to gather a range of responses. The less something varies, the easier it is to capture the range of experience or opinion with a smaller sample.

Qualitative research

As we have seen throughout this and other chapters, qualitative research is so different from quantitative research that different considerations exist in almost all elements of the study, including sample size. Holloway and Wheeler (1996) note that generally qualitative samples consist of fairly small numbers with anything from 4 to 50 participants. They emphasize that in the case of qualitative research it is not the size of the sample that determines the importance of the study. It is possible to find large studies such as the classic study by Kirkham (1989), where she observed 113 labours and interviewed 112 of these women later, having already interviewed 85 women during their pregnancy. It is more usual, however, to find much smaller numbers such as the 9 women included in the study by Ng and Sinclair (2002) that looked at women's experience of planned home birth.

Conducting research

In conducting a research project there are some important decisions that have to be made about the sample. One of the first considerations is to be clear on who or what will comprise the sample. For this to be achieved, unambiguous inclusion and exclusion criteria must be developed.

The type of study to be conducted will influence both the size of the sample and the method of selection. In the case of an experimental approach a probability sampling method will be used with a reasonable sample size in each of the experimental and control groups. If relationships are sought but ethical or practical constraints prevent random allocation, then a quasi-experimental or ex post facto approach may be used.

In survey designs the important decision is the extent to which there is a need to generalize further than the study group. This will influence the choice between probability and non-probability sampling methods. Where probability-sampling methods are required, a sampling frame of all possible candidates for the study is required. This should be as complete as possible to avoid bias.

In surveys that do not require generalizations to be made to the larger population, and for qualitative studies, non-probability methods can be chosen. These are far more flexible and simple, and do not require a sampling frame of individuals.

In terms of sample size, the approach used will dictate whether a large sample of near 100 or above will be required, or whether smaller numbers of ten or even less will be adequate.

When writing up a research report the researcher should clearly specify the details of the sample in the methods section. This should include the rationale behind the inclusion and exclusion criteria, the sampling approach, and the choice of sample size.

Critiquing research

In critiquing research one of the first areas to consider is the extent to which the inclusion and exclusion criteria may reduce or increase bias. What is the rationale given by the researcher for the choice of criteria? Using professional judgement, do those included seem more or less representative as a result of the criteria?

An important aspect is whether the researcher has attempted to generalize further than the sampling criteria would allow. For instance, have statements been made about all women in pregnancy or labour, when the sample consisted of only primigravid women, or excluded those of a certain age, social class, or other social elements?

Was the appropriate sampling method used in the study? The researcher should have provided a clear rationale for the choice of sampling method, and given clear details concerning the process of selecting the sample. This should be examined carefully to ensure that the correct procedures are evident. For example, if the researcher says a random sample was used, can we be sure they do not mean a convenience sample. There should be mention of a table of random numbers or other device if it was truly random. In producing systematic reviews of the literature, studies are evaluated very carefully in terms of the details provided to support the statement that individuals were randomized.

In the case of probability sampling, is a sampling frame mentioned and does it seem complete? Has a non-probability sampling method been used, and has the researcher attempted to generalize to the wider population?

The influence of sample size should also be assessed. In an experimental design was there any problem with the number of individuals dropping out of the study that may have affected the extent to which the groups were comparable at the end of the study?

If the researcher is clearly using a qualitative design, we should expect small numbers. We should still expect some detail on the sample characteristics so that we can judge whether they were in a position to provide information on the phenomena that forms the focus of the study.

The more detail provided on the sample the more able we are to judge the extent to which the researcher has been rigorous in the way the study has been conducted.

Key Points

◆ Research rarely collects data from a total population. Usually research is conducted on a sample taken as representative of a larger group. A sample can consist of people, objects or events.

◆ A sample should be defined in terms of inclusion and exclusion criteria.

◆ Sampling methods vary according to whether the study takes an experimental, survey or qualitative approach. Sampling methods or strategies, can be divided into probability and non-probability methods.

◆ Probability sampling methods allow generalizations to be made from the findings to the larger population. Alternatives include simple random sampling, systematic random sampling, stratified random sampling, proportionate random sampling and cluster sampling. In experimental designs, random allocation is more usual which relates to how individuals are allocated to the experimental and control groups.

◆ Non-probability sampling methods include opportunity or convenience sampling, quota sampling, snowball sampling, and purposive sampling. These are usually used in surveys and qualitative methods.

◆ Although non-probability samples are weaker in design, as it is not possible to say whether the findings are generally applicable, they are easier to apply. In the case of qualitative research, it is not the intention to generalize to a wider population, only to say that certain issues can be identified as relevant when considering a topic.

◆ Sample size is influenced by the nature of the study, the availability of subjects, and factors such as response rate. Experimental studies may be modest in size with 25 to 40 in each group, to quite large numbers such as 100 to 200 or considerably more in each group. Surveys can be modest ranging from around 20 to several hundreds. Qualitative research can be anything from under 10 to usually around 12 to 20. These numbers are only rough guidelines, and should not be interpreted as anything more.

References

Burns N and Grove S (2001) The Practice of Nursing Research: Conduct, Critique, and Utilization (4th edn). Philadelphia: W.B. Saunders.

Hicks C (1996) Undertaking Midwifery Research: A Basic Guide to Design and Analysis. New York: Churchill Livingstone.

Holloway I and Wheeler S (1996) Qualitative Research for Nurses. Oxford: Blackwell.

Kirkham M (1989) Midwives and information giving during labour. In: Robinson S and Thomson A (eds) Midwives, Research and Childbirth. Volume 1. London: Chapman and Hall.

LoBiondo-Wood G and Haber J (2002) Nursing Research: Methods, Critical Appraisal, and Utilization (5th edn). St Louis: Mosby.

Moffat H, Lavender T and Walkinshaw S (2001) Comparing administration of paracetamol for perineal pain. British Journal of Midwifery 9(11): 690–694.

Morse J and Field P (1996) Nursing Research: The application of qualitative approaches (2nd edn). London: Chapman & Hall.

Ng M and Sinclair M (2002) Women's experience of planned home birth: a phenomenological study. RCM Midwives Journal 5(2): 56–59.

Polit D, Beck B and Hungler B (2001) Essentials of Nursing Research: Methods, Appraisal, and Utilization (5th edn). Philadelphia: Lippincott.

Streubert H and Carpenter D (1999) Qualitative Research in Nursing: Advancing the Humanistic Imperative (2nd edn). Philadelphia: Lippincott.

West J, Tuffnell D, Jankowicz D, and McCandlish R (2001) Randomised trials: changing the culture of maternity care. British Journal of Midwifery 9(12): 766–769.

CHAPTER FIFTEEN
The Challenge of the Future

> The last chapter of a novel usually reveals all, and brings the plot to a close. It often has a happy or at least intriguing ending, so that the reader puts down the book with a feeling of contentment, perhaps mixed with a tinge of regret that the characters will no longer be a feature of their life. Non-fiction books are not like that. The aim of this chapter is to emphasize that what has gone before in the previous chapters is only the beginning. This chapter challenges you to continue using the information in this book on an increasingly regular basis as part of your clinical practice. It will also encourage you to make a vital contribution to evidence-based practice. This is the last chapter but it is not goodbye.
>
> To consider the challenge of the future, the relationship between the midwife and research will be examined under two themes: the midwife as the producer of research, and the midwife as the user of research. These will be considered in relation to developments in midwifery research. It is intended that this final chapter should stimulate you to reflect on what you can do now, and in the future, to make best use of the information contained within this book.

Closing the credibility gap

As Soltani et al (2002) observe, one of the major challenges in evidence-based health care is the wide gap between research and practice. More good quality research is available than is used. Although legislation to provide evidence-based practice has started to change the culture of health care, midwives still face problems in playing a prominent role in moving practice forwards, even on the basis of clear research evidence. How can we play a more proactive part in shaping the future of midwifery care, particularly in refocusing on the normality of pregnancy and labour?

If we are to close the credibility gap between research and practice, the first stage is to ensure that all midwives share the same philosophy and understanding that professional knowledge must continually move forwards. To achieve this we must constantly be challenging the basis of our activities and look for new evidence to support clinical decision making. This is summed up by McSherry et al (2002) in regard to nursing as follows:

> *It is no longer acceptable for nurses to base care on ritual and tradition – they must be able to justify the decisions they have made about appropriate care and treatment on the basis of a professional expertise which includes using research evidence to inform practice.*
>
> (p. 1)

This is a serious challenge that relates to midwifery as much as other health care groups. However, if midwifery is to change, it cannot do so without certain factors being present. Mulhall and Le May (1999) suggest that these preconditions include the following:

◆ The availability of appropriate evidence
◆ The critical scrutiny of that evidence for rigour and applicability
◆ The conversion of that evidence into an applied form
◆ The acceptance of the evidence as legitimate, and its use as the basis for changes in managerial or clinical practice.
(p. 9)

This provides a useful checklist to develop a midwifery strategy to achieve these preconditions. There are encouraging signs that progress is already being made. This book has cited a large number of research projects, which would suggest that midwifery does regularly produce research. Bick (2000) also suggests that the emphasis on midwifery-led services, and the development of evidence-based midwifery practice make this an exciting time for research in midwifery. So where is the problem?

The problem is that although the amount of midwifery research has increased, it is still more of a trickle than a stream. There is still a relatively small research 'capital' (Mulhall 1999a) on which to draw. Renfrew and Proctor (2000) highlight the nature of the problem in the following statement:

> Although we have moved far in the past 20 years, it is not far or fast enough for research to underpin all of our practice, or for us to feel secure that research will continue to grow and thrive. We still find that research is patchy and of inconsistent quality.
> (p. 197)

Walsh (2000) echoes this sentiment, observing that despite some robust research over the last 20 years it appears to have had little impact on practice. He suggests this might be part of a general antipathy of many midwives to using research findings. The challenge for the future, then, is to answer the following questions:

◆ Why is there so little midwifery research produced on a regular basis?
◆ Why don't midwives make more use of the available midwifery research?
◆ How can we improve the situation?

Why is there so little midwifery research?

Just as in nursing, research in midwifery is a relatively new phenomenon. The techniques and skills of research are still being refined whilst few role models exist in practice areas to inspire and encourage the number of midwifery researchers to expand. This means that there is a shortfall in the number of midwives with research skills, and a lack of opportunity to practise those skills once acquired. Renfrew and Proctor (2000) reinforce this view and make the following recommendation:

> We need to increase the numbers of midwives involved in generating knowledge, so that knowledge is appropriate to the needs of midwives, women and babies. This will require investment in research training and a career structure which enables midwives to develop in research, as well as stay within a clinical context.
>
> (p. 201)

Fortunately, there are now a large number of courses at Degree and Masters level that feature research on the syllabus. It is disappointing, then, to find that there is an increasing trend to regard offering students an opportunity to carry out research as undesirable at undergraduate, and even postgraduate level. The usual argument is that the numbers involved could lead to the saturation of potential research subjects, although there does not seem to be any evidence to support this. It is also argued that the quality of student research is so poor it is better to have no research than poor research. This argument is sometimes extended to suggest that it is unethical to submit those receiving health care to poor quality student projects. This, however, seems to say something about the standard of academic supervision, rather than the ability of the novice researcher who needs experience to develop research skills and understanding.

The conclusion is that at the moment there is a lack of midwives developing practical skills in carrying out research. It is not the same to get students to produce a literature review or design a research proposal. Although these activities develop useful skills, isolated from the experience of undertaking research they merely serve to produce a new research theory–practice gap.

If more research is to be produced we must develop acceptable ways of acquiring practical data gathering and data analysis skills. We should also remember that under clinical effectiveness, midwives will be asked to carry out audit where research skills and experience would be a considerable advantage.

How can we increase the opportunities midwives have to gain skills in undertaking research? This should take a variety of forms. Schools of Midwifery need to ensure that they provide courses and study programmes where these skills can be accessed. There should also be opportunities for midwives to shadow those undertaking midwifery research, and to gain secondments to research units where these exist. More midwifery research scholarships, such as the RCM Trust Ruth Davis Research Bursary should also be considered for trained staff.

Why don't midwives make more use of research?

According to LoBiondo-Wood and Haber (2002), there is little value in carrying out research unless the findings are used in practice to improve care. Where research is rigorously carried out, why is it not reaching its target audience and influencing practice? The first problem is that the results of research are not always published and therefore become difficult for others to access. This is one of four options examined by French (1999), who suggests that the reasons for the poor take-up of research findings can include any of the following:

◆ Research knowledge does not exist
◆ Research does exist, but not in a format that is acceptable to practitioners
◆ Research does exist, in an acceptable format, but does not reach practitioners
◆ Research does exist, in an acceptable format, but is not wanted. (p. 86)

French (1999) presents evidence to support all of these arguments, which means that if the problem is complex, the solution is also going to be complex. It is therefore unlikely that a single means of solving the problem exists. Nevertheless, it is important to identify local barriers that can be tackled within a broader strategy for achieving research utilization.

What are some of the main barriers to research implementation? If you consider your own clinical area, what prevents you from making a greater use of the available research that could improve care? It is not difficult to propose a list of issues that need to be tackled. Mulhall and Le May (1999) in their research into the difficulties in creating changes in practice in nursing, identified the areas shown in Table 15.1.

Table 15.1   Reasons for not using research evidence (reproduced with permission from Mulhall and Le May 1999, p. 165)

Attitudes	Lack of cooperation
	Lack of motivation
	Fear
	Resistance to change/ritualized practice
Beliefs	Research will not make a difference
	Research data are not appropriate
	Conviction that current practice is OK
Professional relationships	Medical staff block implementation
	Medical staff consider nursing research substandard
	Nursing colleagues are uncooperative
	Senior staff are resistant to change
Educational issues	Unable to access research
	Lack the skills in critical appraisal
	The language of research makes it inaccessible
	Location of libraries
	Theory–practice gap
Organisational issues	Time
	Pressure of workload
	Too much change

Richens (2002) applied this table to her examination of midwives' use of research and added the category of economic issues. These included a lack of resources and not enough staff as further problems. Together, these areas illustrate the many barriers facing midwifery that need to be surmounted if it is to be more research based. Time naturally is a big problem, but easy access to the Internet so that information databases can be accessed is a further problem. Midwives also need to develop skills in using the Web, searching for material and critiquing it once located.

We must also recognize that research implementation takes place within a culture that has traditionally been dominated by medicine. Mulhall (1999b) suggests we need to be aware of what makes certain groups powerful when it comes to influencing policies and procedures, and to develop a more sophisticated approach to analyzing what actions we need to develop. In a similar vein, Walsh (2000) points out the frustrations of the pervasive culture of consultant-led labour wards where midwifery research findings are marginalized within an interventionist environment. We need then, to take account of what Phillips (1986) cited in Polit et al (2001) calls historical 'baggage' whereby groups such as midwives have not always viewed themselves as responsible for driving change forwards based on research results. Midwifery needs to be more research proactive in producing and using research to achieve change. This must be developed together with an increased political awareness of strategies required to influence real decision making at both a clinical and strategic level.

How can we improve the situation?

The suggestions made so far depend on one major development, and that is a research culture that values research as an integral part of clinical decision-making. The starting point for this must be a shared concept of what is meant by research and how it can be used to improve practice. Too many people may well have a negative view of research, and feel it is all jargon and statistics. Maben (1999) highlights this problem in nursing when she suggests the following:

> *Research is fun, interesting and relevant to practice, yet many nurses do not think of it as any one of these things, let alone all three of them!*
> (p. 125)

Similarly, Mulhall (2002) proposes that many practitioners' perception of research is one of a slightly mysterious, difficult and elite activity. These views can dissuade midwives from considering how research can be part of the skills and role of the clinical practitioner. It is essential, as Aslam (2000) notes, that midwives share a positive perception that research is important, and that it must be the foundation of evidence-based practice.

We also need to develop a challenging approach to conventional practice. Richens (2002) highlights the danger of complacency by posing the question 'why do midwives continue to accept and use interventions that cannot be justified?' The answer lies perhaps in a natural desire to remain within a comfort zone of familiar practices and procedures. This can be typified by those who support an attitude of 'if it's not broken, why mend it?' However, as Polit et al (2001) point out, simply maintaining current approaches to practice has its own risks. They suggest that failure to change, especially when based on sound evidence, is costly to ignore for all concerned, including those on the receiving end of care.

We also need to acknowledge the wide variety of research that is essential in developing midwifery knowledge and practice. Mulhall (1999b: 169) has similarly suggested that nursing should resist 'falling under the yoke of an entirely biomedically driven evidence-based agenda'. By this she means that we need to avoid seeing research as only useful if it relates to clinical outcomes demonstrated through a randomized control trial. Although outcomes are a primary concern in midwifery, we also need to take account of other aspects of care, such as how the experience of pregnancy and delivery is perceived by those going through it. There are other legitimate forms of research evidence, such as qualitative research, that more aptly inform some midwifery decisions.

The acceptance of a range of research approaches to underpin evidence-based practice will take a change in culture, and a move away from research being seen as a synonymous with the randomized control trial (RCT). Certainly this is a challenging goal to achieve, but one that must be accomplished if a holistic approach to midwifery is to be realized.

We also need to rethink our attitude towards change, and see it as a fundamental feature of the continued drive towards better care. Understandably, most people's attitude towards change is not neutral. The past has seen many developments that have not made midwifery easier, nor improved the quality of care given to women. This has led to scepticism and distrust towards change. Greenhalgh (2001) notes that management theory literature clearly demonstrates that health professionals will oppose changes that they perceive as threatening their livelihood and income, their self-esteem, sense of competency, and autonomy. Similarly, health professionals have traditionally felt very threatened by change and see suggestions for change as a personal attack on their clinical judgement. We need to find ways in which change can be discussed and examined positively, without it being seen as a personal threat or attack. If we are to achieve this we need, as Mulhall (1999b) suggests, to establish a collaborative and supportive outlook within the clinical area as a whole.

Change is about examining your own individual practice, but it is also much more than this. It is about creating an environment where change is not perceived (as is currently the case) as another imposition from above, an irritation, yet another attempt to undermine expert practice. This will only come through a consciousness-raising exercise and a more free and equal dialogue between the different groups involved in health care provision. Sustained change can only be created through dialogue, reflective practice and liberation.
Mulhall (1999b) p. 175

We need to look, then, at our personal reaction to change and how we can improve our management of it. Change in the work setting is difficult to isolate from the other areas of our life. We are all made up of many different facets and roles, so that a change in one area will inevitably have consequences for other areas. Taylor (1999) provides a constructive analysis of change and amongst many useful suggestions, outlines the following factors that will affect our personal management of change:

- The context of change
- The frame of reference we have for this experience
- The weight of the particular event itself
- What else is going on in our world?
- How far this change is related to the life stage of the individual
- The extent to which the individual has a zone of stability in their personal life (If work is changing, how stable is the pattern of personal relationships, for example, as a way of compensating?)
- The emotional stress of the event and the strain of the process
- The cognitive readjustment necessary to make sense of the process. (p. 166)

This illustrates a far more positive approach to change and recognizes that it may not be a comfortable place to be. This checklist suggests that we need to take a more open systems view of change and consider the impact of change on our total life experience. In any setting then, there is complexity of forces to be met by those responsible for introducing change. This means that an additional skill required if midwifery is to progress is the art of change management. Hunt (1997) sees this very much as understanding and dealing with resistance, and warns that all midwives will have to come face to face with the uncertainty, the fear and the challenge of change.

How can we develop a dynamic research culture in midwifery?

The way ahead lies in more midwives developing research skills, both in carrying out research and in critically analyzing published work. Firstly, under developing research skills, it is important to emphasize that we should not expect every midwife to carry out research. Not everyone has the inclination, motivation, or availability of time to become involved in research. Yet someone needs to do it. Clark (2000) argues very forcibly that we need more and more midwives to undertake research training programmes that will enable individual researchers to develop methodological expertise. We need more midwifery researchers producing high quality research that can inform practice.

How do we develop a research-producing culture? One useful development has been the number of midwives involved in audit. This is only a short step away from research. The two activities are very close, and should be carried out with the same attention to rigour. The similarities are such that the midwife who has become proficient in audit has only to broaden the questions that drive the activity to become a researcher. As audit draws in the main on quantitative approaches, it would be useful to extend the repertoire of skills by undertaking a research course, either as a stand-alone module, or as part of a Degree or Masters course.

More midwives must be encouraged to carry out good research. Hicks (1993) suggests that the reasons for this include the need to maintain professional autonomy and credibility, as midwifery needs to develop a sound research base. She also believes it is important for midwives' own professional development and their credibility as a unique, discrete group. However, the most important reason, also supported by Hicks (1993), is to enhance the quality of care given by the midwife. There is a continuing need for midwifery to avoid complacency and to challenge routine procedures through research activity.

In terms of midwifery developing a culture of using research, this book has already attempted to provide an understanding of the ways in which midwives can become critical readers of research. Although this is a useful asset for the individual, it becomes even more valuable where it contributes to a research culture. This means sharing the results of critiquing with others, firstly, on a small informal basis with colleagues who may also be developing this skill, then, when more experience and confidence has developed, with a larger group of midwives. This can be as part of a small research appreciation group, or as a Journal Club. The latter is seen by Haddock (2002) as a valuable way of reflecting on one's own practice, and considering ways to improve efficiency and effectiveness. The outcome can be a contribution to the work area. Critical reviews of the literature can be undertaken by small groups of midwives as a basis for establishing clinical standards, or as a way of solving clinical problems or simply exploring new techniques and practices.

Both critiquing and reviewing the literature are high-level skills that are developed with guidance and practice. In carrying out these activities, it is also important to use professional knowledge and judgements, and to be creative in the use of the available work. Do not expect to find the perfect answers to the problems facing you. It is often a case of skilfully applying knowledge from one area to suit the needs of a slightly different question, whilst recognizing the possible limitations that may be the inevitable consequence of this.

Clinical effectiveness provides the ideal opportunity to develop a meaningful research culture in midwifery. This should not only improve the use of research, but also place research within the context of professional midwifery practice and the needs and wishes of women. However, this will depend on midwives being proactive and joining together in their clinical area to decide on activities that could benefit from a stronger evidence base. Senior midwives and heads of midwifery will sometimes identify suitable topics that need to be explored. This may result in a working group of staff to examine the literature and develop suitable guidelines that will later need to be audited. This provides a great opportunity to get started and develop suitable skills. This should then lead to those who have been involved suggesting further areas for investigation from their own experience and reflection on practice.

In both situations it is important that criteria are used to assess the suitability of a topic as a clinical effectiveness initiative. The following Box

1. The priority of this topic for midwifery and for the organization
2. The magnitude of the problem (small, medium, large)
3. Applicability to several clinical areas
4. Likelihood of the change to improve quality of care, decrease length of stay, contain costs, or improve satisfaction with service
5. Potential 'landmines' associated with the topic and capability to diffuse them
6. Availability of baseline quality improvement or risk data that will be helpful during evaluation
7. Multidisciplinary nature of the topic and ability to create collaborative relationships to effect the needed changes
8. Interest and commitment of staff to the potential topic.

Box 15.1 Selection criteria for a clinical-effectiveness initiative (reproduced with permission from LoBiondo Wood and Haber 2002 p. 419)

adapted from the work of LoBiondo-Wood and Haber (2002) provides a suitable starting point.

This provides a useful checklist of criteria that can be used to identify possible problem areas in relation to a proposed initiative for change. Such an examination should identify what Polit et al (2001) call the 'implementation potential' of a topic. The point has already been made that change is rarely a neutral activity and many practitioners will feel emotionally attached to certain ways of working and so feel distressed to even think about changing or giving them up.

This section has put forward some simple suggestions for developing a more dynamic research culture in midwifery. There are certain to be more creative alternatives that can be developed. We do have to remember the barriers to change and that the best change may be in the form of a gradual evolution rather than a revolution. In other words, it is better to start in a modest way rather than have high aspirations dashed by a lack of overall support and commitment. It is better to start with a small group of enthusiasts and then work outwards. These suggestions should be used to consolidate and extend the way we think about the midwife's role and developments for the future. An important aspect of this is to balance the science of research with the natural creativity of midwifery. This is a point brought out by Renfrew and Proctor (2000) who make the following suggestion:

A fundamental skill in midwifery is being able to blend both art and science to offer the best care. Being able to integrate knowledge derived from research with the skills of communication, judgement, decision making and hands-on care is the basis of excellent practice.
(p. 195)

Conducting research

The starting point for research is to have a clear question that needs to be answered. The aim of this chapter has been to encourage midwives to think about their part in taking research forward, and one way is by undertaking a project. This does not have to be elaborate, time consuming or costly. Hicks (1993) has pointed out that one possible reason for the reluctance to get involved in research is the misunderstanding that to be of use, research has to be large scale, costly, and of earth-shattering significance. Small-scale projects, she points out, can have equally useful ramifications for clinical practice, policy and resources.

There are so many changes going on in midwifery at the moment that there is no shortage of developments that need to be evaluated. Buggins and Nolan (2000) make a very important suggestion on what needs researching by emphasizing that it should support and involve the needs of women consumers of maternity services.

> *Midwives, however, are unlikely to find themselves at variance with the research agenda set by women and their families, as the agenda is often concerned with issues around satisfaction with the birth, self-care, social support, and the experience of early parenting.*
> (p. 95)

To carry out research successfully, it is important to have support from professional and managerial colleagues. You must possess a reasonable amount of research knowledge and be able to call upon an experienced researcher to provide guidance and, where necessary, supervision. It is always important that the project remains yours and does not become something your supervisor or adviser would really like to do themselves. In research, you also need a great deal of luck. It is fair to say there is never the perfect research project, and you must always expect the unexpected. It is a little like working with technology, if something can go wrong then it usually will. The compensation is that research is a truly exciting activity. Unlike the accusation that researchers only find what they want to find, if you have designed your project rigorously and with the minimum of personal bias, there is no telling what you will find. And that's what makes it fun!

Once your study is complete it must be communicated. Firstly, to managers who may have supported it and, where possible, to those who may have taken part, even if this takes the form of a one page summary, to let them know that their participation contributed to something tangible. If the study was completed rigorously, then whether the results were positive or negative a clear attempt should be made to disseminate it widely. This can be in the form of any or all of the following:

♦ A conference paper
♦ A conference poster
♦ A journal article.

Each has its own format, and serves a different function. A conference paper requires verbal and visual presentation skills, good voice projection, enthusiasm and a willingness to share your work with a group. Make it easy to understand. Use overheads, slides or PowerPoint presentations with key words or phrases and easy to assimilate tables that are neither too small to see, nor too crowded with information. Overheads and slides allow you to talk around them instead of having to read from a carefully prepared script. Prompt cards are a good idea, but avoid a ten-page script if you want to keep your audience awake.

Poster presentations are a good introduction to research presentations, as they expose you to the minimum of intimidation. These depend on visual impact, and gaining the reader's attention. Try and attend a conference first that has a wide variety of posters so that you can gain some good ideas. Don't forget to include your name and address on the poster so people can get in touch with you for more information. Brief summaries of the research that people can take away are a good idea, but again include your name and address. For both conference and poster presentations, business cards, or even compliment slips will be extremely useful, and will save you writing down your address for people in a hurry.

A journal article is one of the best ways to communicate your research to as wide an audience as possible. Mander (1995) suggests that this is crucial to research and should be considered as a stage in the research process itself. Journal articles differ depending on the journal to which you are submitting, as each has its target audience and journal style. Do not submit to more than one journal at a time. It is acceptable to rework your article once published, for another journal, as long as it is not simply a rehash. Focus on a slightly different theme. Don't try to condense a whole dissertation, or long assignment into a 2000-word article, just concentrate on two or three of the main themes. Make the article interesting by thinking of it from the reader's point of view.

If you are new to writing articles, seek the advice of someone who has already published. Co-authorship is also an alternative where you enlist the skills of someone with publishing experience. Always insist on your name going first.

The usual structure for conference papers, posters, or articles is as follows:

♦ Introduction to the focus (what was the problem)?
♦ What does the literature say about it?
♦ What was the aim of your work (the terms of reference)?
♦ How did you go about it (methods and sample)?
♦ What did you find (results)?
♦ What does it all mean (discussion)?
♦ What do you recommend?

Whichever medium is chosen to communicate research findings, it is important to remember your audience, and the reason you are communicating. Do not perpetuate the myth that research is written in gobbledegook. Hardy and Mulhall (1994) emphasize this by warning that the researcher may be tempted to appear 'scientific' by using research terms and concepts that require a great deal of prior knowledge on the part of the recipient. Where technical terms are used in your report, make sure that their meaning is clear to the novice. Remember, you were there once.

Critiquing research

Throughout this book emphasis has been placed on the skill of critiquing. This is a prerequisite for moving the culture of midwifery forwards. Practice is needed in critiquing and each article will present its own challenges. Long (2002) supports this view and suggests the following:

> *Becoming a more critical reader requires a change in approach. We need to interact with the report. Careful and close reading is needed. Prior to deciding on the potential clinical significance or action implication of the findings, we must engage with the way the study was done, the appropriateness of the design, and execution of the study design.*
> (p. 46)

In this final chapter we should think not only of critiquing research but also of undertaking reviews of the literature (see Chapter 5) and implementing the findings where relevant. This may also mean ensuring that staff have the skills or are helped to acquire the skills indicated by the proposed change.

We also need to think about how we can disseminate the critiques and reviews of the literature to contribute to a research culture. Mulhall and Le May (1999) see this as part of a total process where the individual has to face personal challenges as well as environmental ones. They suggest that the factors affecting the success with which the individual may base more of their practice on research includes:

◆ Their education: have they been taught the skills of critical appraisal?
◆ Their ease of access to up-to-date research articles: is the library close at hand?
◆ The amount of time they can allocate to such activities: are they overwhelmed by clinical work?
◆ Their professional position: are they able to suggest and/or make changes to practice?
◆ The atmosphere of the unit/organization where they work: is innovation encouraged and supported?
  (p. 31)

This will not be an easy task. Although clinical effectiveness depends on all those in a clinical area agreeing standards related to key activities, we may have to start small and develop important skills before we work effectively on the bigger picture. At a preliminary stage we should be satisfied with a small group of individuals who can share our enthusiasm. We will not gain the support of everyone. A small successful Journal Club, or research interest group will be more satisfying and beneficial than a large group where only a small number turn up, and you end up doing all the work.

Research folders, and research notice boards are a good way to disseminate information, providing they are regularly updated. Some invited speakers will also stimulate interest, but don't plan them for when most people are on holiday or when there is something else going on. A guest speaker and three people can be embarrassing and hard work. I know; I have been that guest speaker.

Key Points

♦ Midwifery research is now on the point of entering a new era of maturity. The challenge is to increase the amount of quality research produced, critically evaluated and, where appropriate, implemented. The credibility gap between the amount of research produced and the amount put into practice must be reduced. Emphasis must be placed on developing a supportive midwifery research culture for this to happen.

♦ More midwives need to develop the practical skills of undertaking research. There is no shortage of clinical problems that need examining, and new developments that need evaluation. More encouragement is needed for midwives to develop these skills, and support given to undertake research underpinned by an efficient system of funding.

♦ Once complete, midwifery research should be communicated by means of conference papers, conference posters and articles. These should be clear, unambiguous and action orientated, and seen as a crucial part of the research process.

♦ One of the largest areas of deficit is the number of midwives who can critique research articles and produce critical reviews of the literature. When these activities are undertaken they should contribute to the wider research culture of the clinical area as clinical developments or clinical-effectiveness initiatives.

♦ The suggestions made in this chapter require someone to accept the challenge of the future. Let it be you.

References

Aslam R (2000) Research and evidence in midwifery practice. In: Proctor S and Renfrew M (eds) Linking Research and Practice in Midwifery. Edinburgh: Baillière Tindall.

Bick D (2000) Asking questions about practice and using appropriate research methods. In: Proctor S and Refrew M (eds) Linking Research and Practice in Midwifery. Edinburgh: Baillière Tindall.

Buggins E and Nolan M (2000) Involving consumers in research. In: Proctor S and Renfrew M (eds) Linking Research and Practice in Midwifery. Edinburgh: Baillière Tindall.

Clark E (2000) The historical context of research in midwifery. In: Proctor S and Renfrew M (eds) Linking Research and Practice in Midwifery. Edinburgh: Baillière Tindall.

Downe S (2000) Words into action: disseminating and implementing the findings of research. In: Proctor S and Renfrew M (eds) Linking Research and Practice in Midwifery. Edinburgh: Baillière Tindall.

French B (1999) The dissemination of research. In: Mulhall A and Le May A (eds) Nursing Research Dissemination and Implementation. Edinburgh: Churchill Livingstone.

Greenhalgh T (2001) How to Read a Paper: The Basics of Evidence Based Medicine (2nd edn). London: BMJ Books.

Haddock J (2002) Reflective practice and decision-making related to research implementation. In: McSherry R, Simmons M and Abbott P (eds) Evidence-Informed Nursing: A Guide for Clinical Nurses. London: Routledge.

Hardy M and Mulhall A (1994) Nursing research: Theory and Practice. London: Chapman and Hall.

Hicks C (1993) A survey of midwives' attitudes to, and involvement in research: the first stage in identifying the needs for a staff development programme. Midwifery 9(2): 51–62.

Hunt S (1997) The challenge of change in the organisation of midwifery care. In: Kargor I and Hunt S (eds) Challenges in Midwifery Care. Houndmills: Macmillan.

Long A (2002) Critically appraising research studies. In: McSherry R, Simmonds M and Abbot P (eds) Evidence-Informed Nursing: A Guide for Clinical Nurses. London: Routledge.

LoBiondo-Wood G and Haber J (2002). Nursing Research: Methods, Critical Appraisal, and Utilization (5th edn). St Louis: Mosby.

Maben J (1999) Research dissemination and implementation: the role of education. In: Mulhall A and Le May A (eds) Nursing Research Dissemination and Implementation. Edinburgh: Churchill Livingstone.

McSherry R, Simmons M and Abbott P (eds) (2002) Evidence-Informed Nursing: A Guide for Clinical Nurses. London: Routledge.

Mander R (1995) Practising and preaching: confidentiality, anonymity and the researcher. British Journal of Midwifery 3(5): 289–295.

Mulhall A (1999a) A research culture. In: Mulhall A and Le May A (eds) Nursing Research Dissemination and Implementation. Edinburgh: Churchill Livingstone.

Mulhall A (1999b) Creating change in practice. In: Mulhall A and Le May A (eds) Nursing Research Dissemination and Implementation. Edinburgh: Churchill Livingstone.

Mulhall A (2002) Nursing research and nursing practice: an exploration of two different cultures. Intensive and Critical Care Nursing 18(1): 48–55.

Mulhall A and Le May A (eds) (1999) Nursing Research Dissemination and Implementation. Edinburgh: Churchill Livingstone.

Polit D, Beck B and Hungler B (2001) Essentials of Nursing Research: Methods, Appraisal, and Utilization (5th edn). Philadelphia: Lippincott.

Renfrew M and Proctor S (2000) Developing research and evidence-based practice in midwifery – the next 20 years. In: Proctor S and Renfrew M (eds) Linking Research and Practice in Midwifery. Edinburgh: Baillière Tindall.

Richens Y (2002) Are midwives using research evidence in practice? British Journal of Midwifery 10(1): 11–16.

Soltani H, Hampshaw S and Thornton-Jones H (2002) Antenatal screening: turning research into practice. British Journal of Midwifery 10(4): 243–246.

Taylor B (1999) Personal change. In: Hamer S and Collinson G (eds) Achieving Evidence-Based Practice: A Handbook for Practitioners. Edinburgh: Baillière Tindall.

Walsh D (2000) Part six: Limits on pushing and time in the second stage. British Journal of Midwifery 8(10): 604–608.

GLOSSARY OF COMMON RESEARCH TERMS

Abstract: Published reports and dissertations usually begin with an abstract. This is a one or more paragraphs giving a brief, but succinct overview of the study. If you read this, you should be able to establish if the report is relevant for your purposes.

Accidental sampling/sample: See *Convenience sampling*.

Action research: A research design that involved the introduction and evaluation of change. There is no control group, which makes generalizations difficult. However, something is introduced which might make a positive difference to the setting. Its advantage is that it involves those in the setting in deciding what should take place and how. It has a great potential in midwifery practice, but is probably underutilized.

After-only design: Form of experimental design where there is only one measurement taken following the introduction of an intervention. This has the advantage of not building on previous exposure to information or measurements. However, the disadvantage is there is no baseline available to know if there has been any improvement from a previous level. An alternative is the pre-test post-test design where measurements are made both before and after the intervention.

Alternative hypothesis: Although this is known as the alternative, it is the form that is more familiar than its opposite, the null-hypothesis, that suggests there is no difference between the groups under study. The alternative hypothesis sometimes called the scientific hypothesis, is the automatic opposite of the null-hypothesis and predicts that there is a difference between the groups that is unlikely to have happened by chance.

Analysis: The systematic method of making sense of the results of the data gathering by the researcher. This should be accurate, and capable of verification. It provides the answer to the research question.

ANCOVA: Abbreviation of **AN**alysis of **COVA**riance. This is a statistical procedure used to test mean differences among groups on a dependent variable and tries to ensure that other variables (covariates) are not influencing the apparent relationship.

ANOVA: Similar to the above and stands for **AN**alysis **O**f **VA**riance. This tests the mean difference between three or more groups and compares how much variability there is within the groups as well as between them.

Anonymity: An essential principle of ethics where it should not be possible to establish the identity of individuals who have taken part in a study, either from the personal name used or any identifying details given about that individual or setting.

Applied research: Research that seeks to solve a particular problem rather than simply add to our knowledge on a topic or concept.

Audit trail: In qualitative research the detail available to allow the reader to follow (or audit) the way the researcher has moved from individual quotes, or observations, to key categories used to make sense of the findings. This contributes to the credibility of the research.

Auditability: In qualitative research, the judgement that the researcher has provided sufficient detail to allow the reader to follow an audit trial and confirm the researcher's conclusions.

Authenticity: Part of the criteria for assessing the soundness of qualitative research. The researcher must demonstrate that attempts have been made to check the accuracy of the findings by such means as a member's check, that is the participants agree the accuracy of what was recorded, and by the researcher using thick rich descriptions of the way in which the study was conducted and the environments and incidents encountered. These should be sufficient for the reader to feel almost as though they are there, and that they recognize the details as relating to real events and people.

Bar graph: A way of showing the results of quantitative research in the form of blocks which help the reader to visualize differences between elements and the quantities involved. These answer the question 'how much of each element' was found?' They differ from histograms as bar graphs have a space between each bar, as the data are discrete, such as primigravida and multigravida, and not continuous data such as height or weight.

Baseline measurements: These are measurements made before a change or intervention takes place. This acts as a comparison for later measurements. Used in experimental studies as part of the 'before' measurement.

Basic research: The opposite of applied research. The purpose of this type of research is to add to knowledge or theory about a topic or concept.

Before and after designs: A type of experimental design, also known as a pre-test post-test design, where measurements are taken before an intervention and after. This has the advantage of establishing changes from a baseline measure. In some situations, however, it can be a disadvantage as people are sensitized to issues or abilities that may influence the performance on the 'after' part of the measurement. An alternative is the after-only design.

Beneficence: In ethics this relates to the principle of doing only good. In other words, there must be a way in which people are not knowingly put at risk of harm in a study. The 'good' aspect can include not only improvements in physical state, but also psychological and social benefits. This principle ensures that the researcher considers how the study will be of benefit to people.

Blinding: The procedure involved in hiding from those involved in a randomized control trial (RCT) who is receiving which intervention. A single blind study is where the subjects in the trial are unaware of which intervention they are receiving, and double blind is where both the subjects and those measuring outcomes are unaware. This is taken as an element of rigour in RCTs and is sometimes a criterion for the inclusion of studies in a systematic review of the literature. Blinding is not possible in all interventions (e.g. episiotomies, where the intervention is clearly apparent).

Blind study: In experimental designs where the subjects do not know if they are in the experimental group receiving the test treatment, or whether they are in the control group receiving the placebo or alternative to the experimental intervention. Used to overcome the possibility that subjects will behave differently if they know they are receiving the treatment that is presumed to have a beneficial effect on outcomes. Blind studies reduce bias and increases rigour in trials.

Blind review: This does not relate to the conduct of a study, but to the process of publication. It is a system whereby those asked to evaluate the suitability of an article for publication are not given the names of the authors. This reduces the accusation that only certain people's work appears in print. It is designed to ensure fair publishing opportunities where work is chosen on merit, not the name of the author.

Bias: Anything that distorts or affects the study in a way that will alter or influence the accuracy of the findings. Usually relates to an untypical or unrepresentative sample but can relate to other elements. It is not always easy to spot bias, you need to ask 'is there anything about the way the study was conducted which could have had an adverse influence on the accuracy of the findings?'

Bimodal distribution: A statistical description of the distribution of a variable where the data indicate there are two values that occur with equal frequency. Plotted on a graph, a bimodal distribution would be indicated by two peaks.

Bracketing: In qualitative research the researcher is encouraged to identify their own experiences or expectations that may influence their preconceived ideas about the study, and how findings can be interpreted. These are then put aside or 'bracketed' so that they do not unduly influence the way meaning emerges from the findings. There is some controversy over the extent to which this is possible in practice.

Causal relationship: The objective of experimental designs is to establish evidence of a causal relationship between an independent variable (the cause) and a dependent variable (the effect). It is the statistical relationship between two variables where one (the independent variable) has a direct effect on the other (the dependent variable).

Case study: This is an in-depth study of a single individual or location, such as a clinical area, used to develop insights. The generalizability of the results is low as it depends on the representativeness of the individual or location.

CD ROM: This is an abbreviation for Compact Disc Read Only Memory. It refers to databases, usually in a library, that are used as part of the process of reviewing the literature.

Cell: Tables displaying the results of research are often divided into a number of segments or boxes. These are referred to as cells. One of the most frequently encountered tables is the 2×2 table that has four cells, e.g. male, female, yes and no.

Chi-squared test (x^2) (Pronounced 'ki-squared'): In statistics, a non-parametric test which seeks to establish if the difference between the observed results of a categorical variable (e.g. male, female) are statistically different from the expected value, and are unlikely to have happened by chance.

CINAHL: An abbreviation for Cumulative Index Nursing and Allied Health Literature. This is a popular database used to find relevant literature as part of a review of the literature.

Clinical trial: Research approach that tests the effectiveness of a particular clinical intervention in an experimental design. Statistical analysis is used to establish the extent to which differences between treatments could be due to chance factors.

Closed questions: In questionnaires or interviews where the respondent is only provided with certain alternatives from a list from which they can choose their answer. This makes analysis an easy counting job, but may not provided an accurate representation of the respondent's true answer.

Coding: Method of analyzing qualitative data where an identifying name or category heading is given to recurring items or themes running through the findings.

Cohort: In sampling, a total group defined in some way from which data are collected.

Concept definition: The meaning or definition of a concept used by the researcher in the study. This is stated to clarify the meaning and avoid confusion with competing definitions.

Confirmability: Used in qualitative research as part of ensuring the researcher has demonstrated that the findings are accurate, genuine, and a true representation of the processes involved. If the researcher has met the criteria of *auditability, credibility*, and *fittingness*, then confirmability is achieved.

Consent form: Used as part of ethical principles to ensure the researcher can demonstrate that informed consent has been given. Those taking part in the study, or someone acting on their behalf if this is not possible, should sign this. A witness to the signature who is not a health professional may also be required.

Continuous data: A form of data where the measurements flow along a single scale incrementally, such as height, blood pressure, age. The opposite is discrete data, where items fall into distinct groups or categories and do not flow along a numeric scale, e.g. male, female.

Control: An essential feature of experimental design where the researcher is able to have a large degree of control over the design, particularly in regard to variables that might influence the findings of the study.

Control group: In an experimental design, the subjects who receive the usual treatment, or placebo, and not the intervention or form of the independent variable being tested. The results of measurements from the control group are compared with those of an *experimental group* to establish the existence of a cause and effect relationship.

Constant comparative method: In qualitative research this is a method of analyzing the data where comparisons are made with previously noted items or categories to ensure consistency in the method of analysis.

Convenience sampling: Also called **opportunity or accidental sampling**. A non-probability sampling method that uses those who are in the right place at the right time, and are willing to participate. The limitation is that there is little to guarantee they are representative of the total group. However, it is a cheap, quick way of collecting data, and the findings may not be that dissimilar to more expensive probability methods.

Correlation studies: The aim of these is to reveal a clear pattern of association. It does not imply a cause and effect relationship, only that there is a consistent pattern between two variables. An example would be a correlation between breastfeeding mothers and social class. Social class does not cause women to breastfeed; it is merely a pattern or association that is seen to exist between the two. Although the pattern may be reasonably stable, it does not happen in all cases.

Correlation: A statistical technique that searches for a relationship between two variables in a study. A positive correlation means that as one variable increases, so does the other (e.g. height and weight); a negative correlation is where as one variable goes up, the other goes down (e.g. outdoor temperature and weight of clothing).

Covert observation: Where those in an observation study are unaware that the observer is carrying out a study and observing them. The opposite is overt observation where observation is carried out as visible activity. Covert observations can raise ethical concerns as informed consent may not have been received.

Credibility: Used in qualitative research to ensure that the findings are a true representation of what was said, seen or heard. One method of achieving this is to give informants transcripts of interviews or conversations to confirm as accurate. This is called a *member's check* and is a way of demonstrating credibility.

Critique: A balanced assessment of a piece of research that considers not only what is said, but also how the research was conducted in terms of its strengths and limitations.

Cross-sectional study: A survey that looks at a situation at one point in time. Can by used to look at different forms of one group rather than following the same group over time, e.g. women at different points of pregnancy and following delivery. This is more cost effective than a longitudinal study, but may come up with different findings than following the same group through time.

Crossover-study: Form of experimental design where a group receive firstly one intervention, are evaluated and then receive a second intervention and re-evaluated. This can be done with a single group, or more than one group. This holds constant the variable of individual differences between members in different groups. This way the same individual is responding to both interventions and acts as their own control. The biggest problem is the carry-over effect where the benefits of the first intervention may affect the evaluation of the second. Interventions are frequently randomly allocated to individuals to reduce this problem.

Cross-tabulation: One form of presenting a table of results where one variable, such as age is broken down by another variable, e.g. parity.

Data: Used to describe the material collected by a tool of data collection in a study. This is the plural of datum.

Deductive reasoning: This is a method of analysis that starts from general theories or propositions and then examines the specific results that may support these general statements. This approach characterizes quantitative research, particularly experimental designs.

Dependability: Part of the criteria used to assess the authenticity of qualitative research. The researcher must demonstrate that the findings are credible through such mechanisms as prolonged and in-depth data gathering. If *credibility* is established then dependability is said to have been achieved.

Dependent variable: In experimental design, this is the factor that forms the outcome measured in the study, or the 'effect'. The independent variable is the presumed 'cause'. So in a study examining the relationship between information-giving and feelings of control, the feelings of control would be the dependent variable or effect, and the information would be the independent variable, or cause.

Descriptive research: A research approach which seeks to paint a picture of a situation either in numbers, as in quantitative research, or words, as in qualitative research.

Descriptive statistics: One of the two main forms of statistical analysis that attempts to describe a situation in numbers. The second main form of statistics is inferential statistics that allow inferences to be made about the wider population from which the sample is taken.

Design: This is the plan of action followed by the researcher to achieve the goals of the research, e.g. survey design, experimental design.

Directional hypothesis: Also called the research hypothesis, where a clear prediction is made of the expected outcome between two groups in an experimental setting. This form of hypothesis is indicated by the use of such terms as 'greater than', 'smaller than', 'more often than', etc., in relation to the measurements between the two groups of experimental and control. Other forms of hypotheses include *non-directional*, and *null-hypothesis*.

Discrete data: Also called discontinuous data. A form of data where the measurements fall into clearly different categories, in such as clinical areas medical, surgical, neonatal unit, maternity, etc. The opposite is continuous data where the measurements flow from one value to another on one scale incrementally, such as height, blood pressure, age, etc.

Emic perspective: In qualitative research, this looks at things from the perspective of those experiencing it, using their own words. The opposite is the *etic* perspective that is the outsider, or researcher's perspective, found in quantitative research.

Empirical evidence: This refers to the collection of data in the real world involving the senses of sight, touch and hearing, rather than through assumption or abstract development of an argument. Health service research is largely empirical. Empirical evidence is concrete information that has been gathered in the real world to answer a specific question.

Ethics: A code of research practices and principles considered correct. When planning research involving human subjects, the researcher must consider ethical principles including informed consent, anonymity, an estimation of any possible harm, and justice, that is, treating everyone fairly.

Etic: Perspective in qualitative research, this is looking at things from the perspective of the researcher, or outsider. The opposite is the *emic* perspective which is the insider view of things, in their own words.

Ethnography: A type of qualitative research that attempts to uncover the social world of a cultural group, clients, health staff, from the perspective of those in the situation. It has its roots in anthropology and uses the system of trying to understand unfamiliar tribes and applies them to our own situation with sometimes very revealing results. It tends to be undertaken using observation and interviews over a reasonable time period.

Evidence-based practice: A philosophy of encouraging clinical activity to be founded on sound evidence. Research, particularly in the form of randomized control trials, is a highly regarded source of such evidence. It should also take account of professional consensus of opinion and client acceptance. The aim is to follow best practice for each person receiving health care support.

Experimental design: A classic approach to research that aims to establish cause and effect relationships. It usually consists of two groups where an independent variable in the form of an intervention is contrasted with either usual procedures or a placebo. Accurate measurements are made of the dependent variable to establish statistically if any changes could have happened by chance, or whether the independent variable has produced a difference in the dependent variable.

Experimental group: In an experimental design, the subjects who receive the independent variable, or intervention form the experimental group. The results are compared with a *control group*.

Experimental intervention: This is the form of the independent variable introduced into the experimental group in experimental design and not to those in the control group. It is this that is presumed to be the 'cause' in the cause and effect relationship that is the subject of the experiment.

Ex post facto: A research approach used where an experimental approach involving manipulation of the independent variable by the researcher is not possible. It consists of examining groups where the independent variable is already present in the subjects in at least one of the groups, e.g. smoking. Ex post facto literally means 'after the fact'. As it lacks manipulation and control it is not as strong at indicating causal relationships as the experimental design; the findings may be explained by other factors.

Face validity: A 'face value' judgement, often made by an expert, on the likelihood that a method of measurement will produce accurate results. Frequently used in relation to questionnaires and assessment scales.

Feminist research: A research approach that highlights the disadvantages and unsatisfactory situations facing women because they are women, with the intention of improving the situation.

Field notes: Part of data collection in qualitative research. Describes the details and personal thoughts kept by the researcher whilst engaged in a study.

Field research: The opposite of 'laboratory research', where data gathering is carried out in natural, or real life settings.

Findings: Often used as the qualitative equivalent to the quantitative term 'results', meaning the product of data gathering and analysis.

Fittingness: Used in qualitative research to indicate that the findings of the study may well apply to other situations but not in the exact way indicated by the term generalizability.

Fixed alternative questions: In questionnaire design where respondents are given a list of alternatives from which to choose. The opposite is open questions.

Focus groups: Interview design that uses a small group of individuals to talk about their experiences, feelings or views.

Focused interviews: Where the interviewer uses a flexible and informal approach that centres on a broad list of topics or subject headings with a respondent.

Follow-up study: Used to return to respondents after an initial study to discover any changes or outcomes that have developed. This is a separate study from a previous one and not the same as a 'before and after' study.

Forced choice: See *Fixed alternative questions.*

Frequency distribution: In descriptive statistical presentations, the researcher presents the total figure for each of the categories used in the analysis of a question or group of questions. These are presented in the form of a table.

Gatekeeper: In qualitative research used to refer to those in a setting who can control or limit the researcher's access to subjects, settings or events.

Generalizability: In quantitative research, the ability to apply the results of a study to other like situations. This is one of the aims of quantitative research.

Grounded theory: A type of qualitative research where the aim is to produce an explanation, or theory that is 'grounded' in the findings and arises inductively through the researcher's interpretation and analysis. Developed by two Americans; Barny Glaser and Anselm Strauss.

Hawthorne effect: Where the behaviour of individuals in a study may be influenced by the knowledge of their involvement or participation in a study. Similar to the placebo effect, this is a threat to the validity of a study. The name is taken from an American study on worker motivation set in the Hawthorne electrical plant in Chicago.

Histogram: Line drawing used to display numeric results in the shape of a series of blocks. Histograms differ from bar graphs in that the blocks touch, as the data used are continuous not discrete.

Historical research: A research design that looks systematically at past situations or problems, using historical records, objects, diaries and verbal, or visual accounts produced by those who witnessed them.

Hypothesis: In experimental designs, this is the researcher's prediction of what they might find if the theory being tested can be supported. It outlines the relationship between the independent and dependent variables in the study. It can take a number of different forms such as directional, non-directional and 'null'.

Independent variable: In experimental research, this is the cause or intervention that is believed to influence an outcome or dependent variable.

Inductive reasoning or approach: This form of analysis starts with a group of observations or data and on the basis of these, formulates general principles that might explain the patterns or relationships. This form of reasoning is a feature of qualitative research. This is the opposite of *deductive reasoning*, which starts with general principles, and then examines the data to confirm the explanation.

Inferential statistics: One of the two main categories of statistical analysis that attempts to use the numerical results of a study as the basis of reasonably accurate inferences. The second main form of statistics is *descriptive statistics*, which provides a numeric picture of a situation.

Informant: Used to describe someone providing interview data, and has a less manipulated connotation than 'subject'.

Informed consent: An ethical requirement to gain permission from an individual invited to take part in research, based on a full understanding of what will happen, possible advantages and disadvantages, and other relevant details. It is expected that this should be gained in writing.

Institutional Review Board (IRB): The American equivalent of a Research Ethics Committee (REC). Its role is to provide ethical approval for studies.

Instrument: Describes the tool used to collect data in a study. A questionnaire, or assessment scale can be described as an instrument.

Internal validity: The ability of the research design to measure the true effect of the intervention rather than the effect of influences outside the study.

Inter-rater reliability: The extent to which more than one data collector in a study assesses the same outcome, situation or result in an identical way.

Interval measurement: Level of measurement that produces numerical values. Differs from the next category of ratio level in that it does not have an absolute zero.

Interview: Method of collecting data through face-to-face, phone or inter-active method. Can be on a one-to-one or group basis. Interviews vary in structure and depth.

Interview guide: Used in in-depth interviews as a way of providing a broad structure and direction. Takes the form of general questions, topics or subjects that can be referred to in a flexible way. Differs from an interview schedule that is more fixed.

Interview schedule: Fixed list of questions similar to a questionnaire, used in interviews to produced standardized results. Differs from interview guide that is more flexible.

Item: In a Likert scale, used to describe a statement to which the respondent may chose to 'strongly agree' or to 'strongly disagree'.

Judgemental sample: Also more commonly known as a purposive sample. This is a non-probability sampling strategy where those in the study are picked on the basis of the researcher's knowledge of their characteristics that will contribute to a balanced or representative sample.

Justice: The ethical principle that all those involved in research should be treated fairly and equally as human beings.

Key informant: In qualitative research, someone who has a special position in the setting or who has valuable information. Key informants provide the researcher with major insights or details crucial to the study.

Key word: In reviewing the literature, this is the word(s) entered into the database in order to discover what has been published under the topic investigated. Care is needed, as words commonly used may not be the same as those under which suitable articles are stored. American spellings can also be problematic.

Levels of measurement: A categorization of the different properties of numbers. Includes nominal, ordinal, interval and ratio levels. This plays an important part in determining the appropriate statistical tests that may be used with the data collected.

Level of significance: The 'P' or probability level in a study that indicates the extent to which the results could have happened by chance. The minimum level is usually set at '$P < 0.05$' which means that statistically, there has to be less than five in a hundred chance of being wrong if the researcher maintained there was a relationship between the independent and dependent variables in the study.

Likert scale: A method of measuring opinion or attitude by asking respondents to 'strongly agree' to 'strongly disagree' with a list of statements or 'items' in an interview on questionnaire. This, usually five point scale is named after the American Renis Likert who developed the technique.

Limitations: All studies have their weaknesses. The researcher should identify those that may affect the outcome of the study and the interpretation of the results. This is usually found at the start of the discussion section.

Literature review: An essential aspect of research studies where the researcher places their study within the context of what is already known about the topic and the recent research that has been conducted on it. This should be critical in nature, and not simply a summary of previous work. Reviews of the literature, especially in their more systematic form, also play an important role in evidence-based practice and in producing standards for audit.

Lived experience: In phenomenological research, an attempt to understand a situation or condition through the eyes of those experiencing it, so we can gain insights and understanding.

Longitudinal study: A type of research that follows a group of individuals over a long period of time to gain an understanding or measurement of any long-term changes, experiences or effects of a variable. Can take the form of a *panel study* where the same people are followed over time, or a *trend study* where different people from the same population are included at different points of time. The time period may range from weeks or months, to years.

Manipulation: One of the features of experimental design is that the researcher must make a change in the situation or to the subjects in the study. This is usually the introduction of the independent variable, or intervention.

Matching: A method of sampling in experimental design where individuals are matched by the researcher in terms of their possession of key characteristics which may have an undue influence or confounding effect on the study. The aim is to divide those with possible confounding attributes such as age, sex, parity equally between the different study groups so that the groups can be compared fairly. This reduces the effect of the confounding characteristic on the outcome as it will affect each group equally.

Methodology or method: The overall design followed by a researcher in carrying out their research, as in *survey method*, or *experimental method*. Each method will follow certain principles, and will be carried out in a series of steps. Methodology is also used in a more conceptual sense in relation to the study of research procedures. In everyday use it is used as a heading in research reports under which the details of how the research was conducted are presented for scrutiny.

Maturation: One of the threats to the validity of an experimental design, where the outcome could be influenced by changes to the individual, either physically or mentally, over the course of the measurement period.

Mean: The statistical term for an average. It relates to what is typical in the group and is part of a series of measures called *measures of central tendency*.

Measure of central tendency: A statistical term for the result of a procedure that attempts to establish a typical single value from a set of numbers. We usually talk about an average, but there are three alternative measures; the *mean*, *mode* and *median*. Each of these can produce a very different result because of the way in which they are calculated.

Median: a measure of central tendency or 'average' in a set of results that identifies the value of a numbers which is midway along a set of numbers which have been put in order from smallest to largest. Fifty per cent of the other values will be above that number and 50% below it. It is a stable measurement and is not unduly influenced by numbers that may be rare, or untypically large or small in the set.

MEDLINE: A computerized database of medical journal articles.

Member check: In qualitative research, the process of increasing credibility by getting those who provided data to check it for accuracy.

Meta-analysis: A method of combining the results of a number of studies on the same topic, carried out in similar ways in order to increase the total size of the study sample. If successful, this can increase the accuracy of the statistical procedures carried out on the data, and so increase the value of the prediction based on the combined outcomes. There are many difficulties in this procedure due to hidden variations and biases in the way different studies have been conducted.

Mode: A measure of central tendency or 'average' and identifies the value of the unit that appears most often in a set of numbers or values. It is not a very good indicator of what is typical in a set of numbers. If two numbers appear in a set the same number of times they form a *bi-modal distribution*. If several numbers appear the same number of times, it is known as a *multi-modal distribution*.

Mortality: In experimental designs, this refers to those who for one reason or another (not necessarily death) left the study. If there is a high mortality rate in one or more of the groups, those remaining in a study may no longer produce a typical group, or allow a reasonable comparison between groups.

Naturalistic study: Used as an alternative description for qualitative research methods, where there is no attempt to control or manipulate, and the study takes places in a normal or natural setting rather than a carefully controlled laboratory setting.

Nominal data: This is the most basic of the levels of measurement and relates to numbers that do not have a value in relation to quantity, but merely label a category with a number, e.g. primagravida = 1, multigravida = 2. It is not possible to carry out statistical procedures on nominal data apart from producing their frequency distribution.

Non-directional hypothesis: Here a clear prediction is not made of the expected outcome between two groups in an experimental setting, only that a difference will be found. Unlike directional hypotheses that use such terms as 'greater than', 'smaller than', 'more often than', etc., in relation to the outcomes between the experimental and control group, non-directional hypotheses merely say there will be a difference. The nature of the difference and in which group it will be found is not stated.

Non-equivalent experimental designs: This indicates that those in the study have not been randomly allocated to the experimental or control group. This means that it is not possible to be certain that any differences are purely due to the independent variable; differences between those in the two groups could have influenced the outcomes.

Non-experimental design: A study where the researcher does not introduce a variable and is not looking for a cause and effect relationship. It should not be inferred that research in this category is less worthy than experimental research, only that the intentions are different.

Non-maleficence: The ethical principle to do no harm in a study. This is one of the most powerful principles of ethical considerations.

Non-parametric statistics: A collection of statistical techniques that do not require the strict criteria of parametric statistics and so can be carried out more easily. The results are not as widely accepted, or as accurate as those in the parametric category.

Non-probability sampling methods: A collection of frequently used methods of selecting the sample in a study that includes opportunity/accidental, quota, and purposive sampling strategies. It is not possible to say with any certainty how typical those selected are of the larger population using any of these methods. Their advantage is that they are relatively easy to apply.

Non-significant result: This does not mean that the results of the research are not important, it means that in the case of a randomized control trial the 'P value' is too large to rule out the element of chance and therefore the null-hypothesis must be accepted. In other words, there was no real difference between the results of the groups involved.

Normal distribution: This relates to a statistical pattern of the distribution of some variables such as height, blood pressure etc. If data on this variable were plotted on a graph for a sample group, it should produce a bell shaped curve where most people are close to the mean, and others are in equal proportion on either side of the mean. In a normal distribution the mean, mode and median all have the same value and graphically would be a single line dropping down from the apex of the frequency curve. A normal distribution allows the use of parametric statistical tests making this an important statistical concept.

Null-hypothesis: This is the hypothesis of no difference, that is, it predicts that there will be no statistically significant differences between the groups in the experiment. It is also called the statistical hypothesis. It is expressed in this way because it is easier to reject the null-hypothesis, than it is to accept its opposite, the research hypothesis, which predicts a direction between the dependent and independent variable. However, if the null-hypothesis is rejected, it leads to the automatic acceptance of the research or directional hypothesis.

Nuremberg Code: Ethical principles originally applied to experimental research on humans. Designed to prevent inappropriate and dangerous research by protecting those involved. Based on ten principles, including informed consent.

Observation: A method of collecting research data through visible means, using either the eye or a camera. This can be structured in the form of quantitative checklists, or unstructured, in the form of qualitative participant or non-participant observation.

One-tailed hypothesis: Also called a directional hypothesis, this predicts a difference between two groups in the study and is indicated by the use of such words as 'more than' or 'less than'.

Open coding: The method of qualitative analysis where codes are given to the categories identified in the data.

Open (ended) questions: In questionnaire design, or interviews where the respondent is encouraged to provide their own response rather than having alternatives to choose from, as in fixed choice alternatives.

Operational definition: The way in which the researcher intends to measure or make operational the variables under study.

Opportunity sampling: See *Convenience sampling.*

Ordinal level of measurement: The category that follows nominal data. Here, the numbers used relate to the position or order of the items in the set. As with nominal data, there are severe restrictions on the statistical procedures that can be carried out on them. Examples include Likert scales that go in order from 'strongly disagree' to 'strongly agree'.

Outliers: In a set of numbers, these are the values at the extreme ends of a distribution that are not necessarily typical of the others in the set.

Overt observation: Where the research activities of an observer are clearly visible and known by those involved to be taking place. The opposite of covert observation, where those in the setting do not know that they are being observed.

'P' value: This is the indicator that the researcher has statistically tested the results, particularly in randomized control trials, to establish the 'probability' that the differences could be due to chance, and not the intervention. The most common values used to indicate that the results are unlikely to have happened by chance are, in increasing size of certainty that the results are real differences – $P < 0.05, 0.01, 0.001$.

Panel design: This kind of longitudinal study takes the form of a survey where the same people are approached for information at two or more points over time. This provides information on how people variables, or experiences change over time.

Paradigm: This is a distinct way of looking at the world around us and aspects of it that colours all aspects of our understanding; it is a 'world view'. So obstetrics and medicine have been characterized as having a very different view of the world compared to midwifery and nursing.

Participant observer: Where the researcher observes whilst carrying out similar activities in the setting as those being observed.

Phenomenology: A qualitative approach that seeks to uncover the 'lived experience' of people in a particular setting or with a particular condition.

Physiological measurement: A precise way of measuring some physiological factor or outcome, e.g. temperature taking or blood pressure monitoring.

Pilot study: A small-scale test to ensure that the tool of data collection is reliable and that there are no unforeseen or unanticipated practical difficulties in following the intended method. The pilot is very much like a dress rehearsal and is an indication of rigour. The flexible nature of qualitative research means that pilots are mainly a feature of quantitative research than qualitative.

Placebo effect: The power of suggestion in drug trials where the belief in the effectiveness of a drug can produce perceived positive outcomes reported by subjects. To reduce this, a non-active drug or treatment is used to act as a measure against the drug or procedure being tested.

Population: A clearly defined group who share common characteristics as specified by the researcher.

Power calculation: Statistical procedure to calculate the size of a sample needed in a randomized control trial to ensure that the statistical calculations are sensitive and accurate.

Primary sources: In a review of the literature where the researcher consults the original authors and studies, and does not depend on secondary sources, which are accounts of them by other authors.

Probability sampling methods: A collection of strategies for selecting a sample from a population that gives a reasonably representative group. Strategies include, simple random sampling, stratified sampling, proportionate sampling, and cluster sampling methods. A number of sophisticated statistical techniques can be used on such samples.

Probing: In interviewing, a way of gaining more in-depth data by asking further questions to elaborate on points. This is not the same as prompting, where the interviewer offers a possible answer accepted by the respondent, although it may be inaccurate.

Proportionate random sampling: A method of ensuring that important subgroups in the sample are in the same proportions as those in the main population. This reduces the risk of bias through uneven sized subgroups who might make a difference to the overall results.

Prospective study: A study where the data lies in the future at the start of the research. Newly occurring data are then collected as the study progresses. This is the opposite of a retrospective study, where the data already exist when the study is set up. Prospective studies have the advantage of greater control by the researcher, and therefore greater accuracy.

Purposive sampling: Also called a judgemental sample. Sampling strategy that hand-picks items or people on the basis of the researcher's prior knowledge of them. Despite sounding as though there is an element of bias here, this type of sample can produce a typical or representative sample.

Qualitative research: Broad heading for a number of approaches that are not so much concerned with numerical accuracy and the need to control or predict, but rather the need for insight and understanding. The findings are in the form of words and descriptions rather than numbers.

Quantitative research: Broad heading for a number of approaches to data gathering that produce numeric results. The concerns of this type of research centre on accuracy, the ability to generalize and to control and predict situations.

Quasi-experimental design: This looks like an experimental study in that the researcher introduces an independent variable, but it uses groups that have not been randomly allocated. This means that the outcome may be due to factors other than the independent variable. However, there are situations where random allocation may not be possible.

Questionnaire: Popular way of collecting research data that consists of respondents writing answers to a written set of questions and returning this to the researcher. The anonymity of this process can be both an advantage and disadvantage.

Quota sampling: A non-parametric sampling strategy often used by market researchers where the researcher predetermines how many in the sample they will recruit with certain characteristics such as age or social class grouping. Once a particular quota is full, emphasis is placed on others that have not been completed.

Random allocation: The method of allocating those in a trial to the experimental and control group so that everyone has an equal chance of ending up in either group. Those in a study may well not be randomly selected from the population, but are the result of recruitment.

Random selection: This ensures that each person in a total population has an equal chance of being selected for study. Where data are gathered from everyone selected, the findings should be reasonably accurate and representative of the population as a whole. A number of statistical tests assume data are taken from a random selection of the population.

Randomization: The technique of randomly allocating someone to either the experimental or control group. This usually involves computer generated random numbers, or tables of random numbers, and sampling frames, or lists of those to be allocated. Other techniques, such as picking names out of a hat or using the last digits on a medical record are less well accepted as achieving a high level of randomization.

Reliability: The accuracy of the tool of data collection. This is usually subject to a number of tests to ensure consistency. A pilot study will also be used to examine the reliability of the tool of data collection unless a well-used tool is applied.

Replication study: A design based on a study that has previously been carried out to confirm the findings of the first. Can take a number of different forms, including replication of the sampling design, the tool of data collection and other testing procedures.

Research: Extending knowledge and understanding through the systematic collection of information that answers a specific question objectively and as accurately as possible.

Research based practice: The approach to clinical activity that bases decision making on the basis of sound research evidence.

Research proposal: An outline of an intended piece of research used to gain ethical approval, permission or funding. It also allows the researcher to think through the whole process and identify any weak areas.

Research question: This is the element that structures the research process, particularly data collection. The results of a study should answer this question.

Respect for persons: Part of the ethical code that sees individuals as autonomous and therefore the need to be given the freedom to determine whether or not to participate in research.

Respondent: Term to describe someone taking part in a study, often used in relation to questionnaires and interviews.

Response rate: The percentage of those returning a questionnaire or agreeing to be interviewed out of those approached.

Results: Usually applied to the numeric findings of a study produced by data collection.

Retrospective study: A study in which the data already exist when the study is set up. These data cannot be influenced by the researcher, which reduces bias. The disadvantage is the lack of control the researcher has on the quality of the data. The alternative is a prospective study.

Review of the literature: See *Literature review*.

Rigour: The extent to which the researcher has actively sought to carry out the study to a high standard. This includes identifying possible pitfalls in the design of the study and reducing their effect as much as possible. The end result should be a study that is as accurate and professional as is possible.

Risk versus benefit ratio: Ethical principle of assessing whether the risks inherent in the study design are outweighed by possible benefits. These should be made known to those asked to take part in a study, particularly where the risks are significant or of an unknown magnitude.

Sample: A section of a defined population used in a study to provide data.

Sampling frame: A list of all those who are eligible to be included in a study according to the inclusion/exclusion criteria. All those in the list are numbered and using a table of random numbers or computer-generated numbers, the researcher draws a predetermined set of numbers, these are then matched against those in the sampling frame to provide the names of those randomly selected.

Sampling strategy: Also referred to as a sampling plan. The choice of method used to select a sample for data collection.

Saturation: In qualitative research, the point at which no new analytical categories are arising from the data analysis, so the researcher stops data collection.

Scientific approach: This is an ordered and objective method of collecting information in such a way as to provide verifiable data. Developed from the natural sciences, such as physics and chemistry, this approach has now been applied to human behaviour on the assumption that we are subject to similar constant patterns and influences. Those who favour a more humanistic approach, such as that of qualitative research, dispute this.

Secondary source: In reviewing the literature, where an author's original work is not consulted, only the work as cited, or outlined, by another author. There are dangers with this as the primary source could be misquoted, or vital information omitted.

Selection bias: Where the sampling strategy used has not resulted in a representative group.

Self-report: Method of data collection that consists of asking people to provide information about themselves, such as in questionnaires, interviews or diaries. Built on the assumption that what people say they do is accurate, which may not always be the case.

Seminal study: Description of a study that was the first to tackle a topic and has become a 'classic'.

Simple random sample: A sampling strategy where everyone or every item has an equal chance of being selected. Requires a sampling frame and a table of random numbers or computer-generated random numbers.

Snowball sampling: Also known as 'chain', 'nominated' or 'network' sampling. A sampling strategy used in qualitative research when it is difficult to identify or locate suitable candidates for the study. The procedure depends on finding some appropriate members, and then asking them for the names of contacts who might be willing to take part. The disadvantage is that as the nominated people will be socially close to the individual the resultant sample may not be representative of the wider group.

Social desirability: In surveys where individuals may answer inaccurately because they want to be seen in a good light.

Stability: Refers to a tool of data collection that is consistent in its ability to provide accurate measurements.

Standard deviation: In statistics, a measure of the average distance of each unit in the study from the mean value.

Stratified random sampling: Method of dividing the sampling frame into appropriate subgroups and drawing the sample from within each one.

Statistical significance: The extent to which the results of a study could have happened by chance rather than the result of an intervention or independent variable. This is indicated by the 'P' value.

Structured interview: Type of interview that has a high degree of structure. Basically, the researcher reads from a questionnaire (called an interview schedule) and writes down the answers. The advantage is that people can be more ready to answer this format than getting around to completing and returning a questionnaire. It also makes the answers more easily comparable with the minimum of coding. The disadvantage is respondents can only follow the line of questioning and wording laid down in the schedule.

Subject: Used to refer to someone in a study.

Survey: A research design that uses mainly questionnaires or interviews to collect descriptive data from a reasonably large sample.

Systematic sampling: Method of numbering all possible units in a sampling frame and then choosing units at a set interval, such as every 10th, to ensure that the entire range of the sample is included.

***t*-test**: Statistical test that compares the means of two groups to establish if any differences between them could have happened by chance.

Terms of reference: The clearly stated aim of a study that guides and provides focus for the research activity.

Theory: In quantitative research, the set of ideas about a situation that guides the construction of a study and its analysis. Hypotheses are developed from theories.

Thick data: In qualitative research where the researcher has provided a great deal of descriptive detail to allow the reader to feel as though they are there, or that will allow them to relate to what is going on.

Transferability: Also called fittingness. In qualitative research the likelihood that the findings could provide insights into other situations.

Trend study: This type of longitudinal study examines different groups of people from the same population at different times to identify any changes in the variable under study. This can include attitudes, experiences, as well as physical, psychological or social changes.

Triangulation: The use of more than one method of data collection in the same study in an attempt to produce more accurate information or understanding.

Trustworthiness: In qualitative research, one of the criteria used in establishing the authenticity and accuracy of the information presented. Can be compared to the concepts of reliability and validity in quantitative research.

Two-tailed hypothesis: Also called a non-directional hypothesis, this predicts a difference between two groups in the study but does not indicate in which direction. It simply states there will be a difference. The wording of the hypothesis in terms of one or two tailed is important when it comes to interpreting the statistical results, as the level of probability does vary between the two.

Unstructured interviews: In qualitative research used as a way of gaining an insight into a situation from the other person's perspective without enforcing the researcher's point of view on the situation. Broad questions and probing are used where necessary to maintain the flow of ideas.

Variable: This is the item or 'thing' that forms the focus of the researcher's attention. Called variables because they vary in some way, e.g. temperature, pulse, age, gender, satisfaction with care received, level of depression.

Validity: The extent to which a tool of data collection has produced what it was intended to produce.

Vignette: Used in questionnaires or interviews. Takes the form of a story, pen portrait of scenario on which the respondents answer questions to reveal their attitude, knowledge or behaviour.

Visual Analogue Scale (VAS): Measuring instrument in the form of a straight line. Respondents indicate their location between the two points on the line, e.g. Most pain ever felt/No pain, extreme anxiety/No anxiety. The points on the scale are given numerical values to allow for statistical processing.

Vulnerable subjects: In ethical considerations, those people who are especially at risk and may not be in a position to give true informed consent, e.g. women in painful labour asked to provide consent to a procedure to which they would not agree in normal circumstances. Other vulnerable groups include children, those who are distressed, those with mental health problems, those with language difficulties and the unconscious.

Website: Computer-accessed location of information on the world wide web (www).

Index

Numbers in **bold** refer to boxes, figures and tables; numbers in *italics* refer to glossary entries